PRAISE FOR A HEART FOR RUNNING

Plot/Idea: McDonnell's perseverance is contagious. His honest approach to his process will inspire others to get off the couch and hit the pavement. While we often think of those that are ranked athletes as people who are physically gifted in some way, McDonnell proves that this is not the case with his compelling story and approach to his hard work.

Prose: McDonnell's compelling story is easy to read and highly inspirational. His encouraging personality shines through his writing.

Originality: *A Heart for Running* succeeds in becoming more than a story about one athlete's journey. This is a book about how running saved the author's life. His refusal to give in to self-doubt will uplift readers.

Character/Execution: The level of detail McDonnell offers--notably, about his training schedule and techniques--proves to be a benefit for readers aspiring to challenge themselves physically.

- THE BOOKLIFE PRIZE

"An amazing read, relatable, thought provoking and lessons for us all to remember what is truly important!"

"A Heart for Running is an emotional rollercoaster, and you feel every single moment with John. Running quite literally saved his life and his story is an inspiration and a beacon of hope for us all."

A HEART FOR RUNNING

A HEART FOR RUNNING

HOW RUNNING SAVED MY LIFE

JOHN MCDONNELL

First published in 2022 by Greative Books Publishing, Ltd.

Grogey Road

Fivemiletown

Tyrone

BT750NT

ISBN Ebook: 978-1-3999-4136-5

ISBN Paperback: 978-1-3999-4138-9

ISBN Hardcover: 978-1-3999-4137-2

This book is dedicated to my wife Roisin and our four adult children, Owen, Catraoine, Aidan and Daniel. You are all my inspiration and make every day a better day.

Seek help when you need it.
You will never be abandoned by
those who truly care,
and you might be surprised
by who those people are.

CONTENTS

INTRODUCTION

Why is it that many of us don't look to improve our lives until we face a personal crisis? We get caught in an unconscious cycle of waking to an obnoxious alarm early in the morning. We hit the snooze button and get an extra nine or ten minutes of sleep before hitting the snooze button again. We spent another restless night tossing and turning in the bed. Disproportionately negative thoughts about problems we've had at work kept a peaceful night's rest beyond our reach once again. After reaching the point where it just won't be physically possible to both spend another minute under the duvet and make it to work on time, we reluctantly remove ourselves and stumble to the bathroom for an all too brief shower. Even there, we try to get that extra 30 seconds of comfort under the stream of hot water, where we find sanctuary from the upcoming horrors of another tedious workday. We rush to get dressed, possibly grab something quick to eat and sprint out the door in order to arrive, just in time, at work. We switch our minds into work-mode and buckle down to survive the day, putting out the fires as they arise. We realise that those problems we were anxious about, the cause of those lost hours of sleep the night before, weren't nearly as bad as we thought. Our brains have the tendency to see the worst in each situation, particularly when we are left alone with our thoughts. Dull and dreary, the day drags on, with much of our time wasted as we attend useless meeting after useless meeting. We get through our tasks, all the while watching the clock and wishing it would tick just that little tock faster and take us to the conclusion of the day.

We do this day after day as the week creeps forward to what we are all working towards: Friday afternoon and our two-day release into the weekend. We take our two or three weeks of holidays every year, but these days, we have our smartphones and emails and we don't ever seem to create any separation from our job. Month in, month out, year after year, time moves on. We had great intentions when we started this career, we thought we'd love to work in this field, but reality kicks in after a few years and it's the same as any other job. Maybe, if things are really unpleasant, we will get off our ass and start a job search, but that is difficult too and there's always *the devil you know,* and all that. Unless we are really motivated to move, we stick around in our current situation, take home our adequate pay cheque every week or month and get our annual pay rise of 2%, if we are lucky. Eventually, we all come to the realisation that we missed out on life as it galloped past us in the blink of an eye. We've been stressing and fretting on some company's behalf. We've wasted all our time doing things for other people who would replace us in a heartbeat if we were no longer there. Among the list of regrets from people on their deathbeds, there is a list that comes up over and over again. Here are a few that resonated with me:

- I wish I had let myself be happier.
- I wish I hadn't worked so hard.
- I wish I took better care of my body
- I wish I'd had the courage to live a life true to myself, not the life others expected of me.

Why don't we take the time to look after ourselves earlier on in life and pursue our passions? Why aren't we taught how to live happier? After all, if we did those things, we would be more productive and have a richer and fulfilling life. Had I realised there were so many things that I could have been doing, and not doing, that would have helped me focus more on myself and in-turn be a better husband, father, and friend, I would have done it many years ago. It took suffering a life critical event to get me to appreciate my mortality more clearly. Fortunately for me, it happened when I was old enough to appreciate what I have and still young enough to change the direction I was travelling. I had to reach the low point in my life before I began taking steps, baby steps at first, towards this type of introspection.

I set out to write a story about running and how it helped me recover from a stroke and subsequent heart surgery. My journey since February 2017 hasn't just been a physical recovery, but the knock-on mental challenges I've faced have been far more difficult. I've made huge strides in my mental health since experiencing post-stroke depression, but it has been a struggle, and continues to be, probably for the remainder of my days. I need to constantly keep my focus on the progress I've made in order to prevent a backwards slide to some of the darker places I've been. Although I get down now and again, I now have tools and techniques in my arsenal to work my way back out of it. Running has a major part to play in all of that. My love for the sport was ignited fairly late, in my forties. Since that time it has made me a better person and I have no doubt it saved my life.

CHAPTER 1
IT'S NEVER ONLY A 5K

THERE IS AN UNUSUALLY blue sky on the morning of August 20, 2010, when my wife Roisin and I arrive at the Peace Link in Clones, County Monaghan. We're thirty minutes early for the Clones 5k. We nervously pay our entrance fee and collect our race numbers before heading back to the car to get ready. Maybe it is because it was our first race ever, but my hands are shaking with anxiety and possibly some tiny shred of excitement. I've only ever seen people running in a race, I've never had to pin a number to my own shirt before. It shouldn't feel this awkward, but I fumble with the safety pins. With about five minutes to go, we see the general horde of people with their own numbers, pinned on much straighter than ours, heading in the same direction, so we join in the mass migration.

On the start line I take a good look at the other runners. There are all kinds of people of every age, shape and size. We are just two more, although we feel like fish out of water. Me, with my white cotton Fruit of the Loom t-shirt, baggy cotton shorts and white socks more suited for a 1980's tennis player than a modern runner. The athletes near the front are all doing stretches or running up and down the road, apparently getting loose for what is about to happen in just minutes. All of those doing these extra exercises look like *actual* runners. They have obviously done this before as they make their way back behind the start line and share a few laughs with each other. I'm not even considering smiling. I'm more or less just trying hard to not have an accident in my shorts in front of all these people.

The organisers go over the course and the places we all need to keep an eye out for potential hazards. They advise us on traffic and explain that we shouldn't be wearing headphones, blah, blah, blah… I can't honestly say I am aware of what they are saying. Scanning the field, it is glaringly obvious that some of these people are going to be lightning fast. Especially those wearing the vests sporting the name of their running club and wearing fancy trainers of outlandish colours.

The time has come. Three, two, one. The starter blows his whistle loudly and we are off. The race starts on a slight down-hill before it flattens out and hits a more undulating section of the course. Roisin and I started somewhere in the middle of the pack and she, having been training a little longer than I had, got out in front of me and found some space on the narrow road.

I know I can run the distance because I had managed it leading up to this point, so I go as hard as I can manage. However, there is a big difference between running and racing. I had been running as a means to lose girth around my middle, not to become a faster runner. There is a young girl just in front of me, maybe thirteen years old or so. As a forty-two year old, I'm not doing so bad keeping up with a thirteen year old, right? But this is gruelling. At the 1k sign I'm already feeling awful and I still have 80% more to do!

I remember from my training that by slowing down my pace, I can cover longer distances, so when the route turns left onto a flat section I settle into a slightly more agreeable pace, but only just slightly. I still want to puke my guts out. My lungs are still burning and my legs haven't experienced a workout like this in years. I hit 2k and my brain is telling me there is 3k to go, that's just over half the course ahead of me. I can do this. I can see Roisin still a little ahead and looking a lot better than I feel. "I really hate this," I think to myself. I am starting to seriously question my life choices.

I pass the 3k point before I turn left once again and look up at what appears to be a mountain in front of me. That is an exaggeration, but it is such an intimidating sight. Roisin is well in front of me now, but I've managed to get in front of my teenage competitor. "Just put one foot in front of the other. Just keep going. Don't stop! Do not walk! Keep running! Holy sweet mother of Peter, what the f*@k was I thinking!" all played on an agitated loop through my mind. My legs and my lungs weren't meant for this. The human body hasn't been required to move like this since we roamed the African plains and were being chased by hungry predators. The crest of the hill is in view as is the 4k signpost. If I can just get to the top, there is a glorious downhill and I'll only have 1k to go. A beautiful, lovely, long-awaited downhill, oh wherefore art thou, downhill?

It seems like it is two miles to the top and is taking three days to reach the 4k mark, but I'm there and now I only have a little further until this torture session is over. This is the worst thing I've ever decided to do. Why would anyone pay money to do this? I hate every single, tiny, little thing to do with this experience. I feel worse than I've ever felt in my life and I've been to insurance conferences. I not only feel sick but also disappointed in my own stupidity in thinking this might be a good idea. I'm smarter than this and when this is over, I will need to seriously rethink my future if I was capable of making such a bad decision.

On the downhill now, my quads are taking a pounding and my lungs feel like they can't get enough air. If only I could take in oxygen through my ears. Oh, and I still want to lose my breakfast. The brain is working overtime with thoughts like, "What would it look like if I fell? Can I die from running downhill?"

Down, down, down and then I turn right into the Peace Link Parking lot. I see the finish line. I can *actually* see the finish line. I find a small burst of energy from somewhere and pick up the pace, just a tiny bit, but I did speed up, didn't I? I cross over the finish line and start to walk. I'm handed a medal. Someone else hands me a bottle of water. Another volunteer points me in the direction of banana boxes and asks me to keep moving. Just walk or crawl, but get out of the finish area. All I want to do is sit my ass down and let my legs recover, but I get out of the way and move to the side where all the other finishers are having their water and bananas and smiling, laughing like this was fun. I finished in a respectable time for a first timer at just over 29 minutes.

Roisin finished 10 seconds ahead of me. She greets me with a hug and we congratulate each other for completing this ridiculous thing. We hold each other up, preventing a collapse. We did it! We ran our first 5k race and survived. After sitting down for just two short minutes we start to see a different perspective on things. Smiles adorn our faces and that rush of endorphins hits our brains. I lean over to Roisin and say, "Wow, we are pretty awesome. I can't believe we did this without stopping. This is amazing and we need to do it again, like soon. Where is the next one?"

One's first 5k is a big achievement, but if you are a seasoned runner it may not sound like a lot. Endurance athletes often say they "*only* ran 5k today," but 5k is a long way to run, especially non-stop, when you're starting out. Even today, having run much further, it is never *only* a 5k!

CHAPTER 2
BORN IN THE USA

I WAS BORN on Halloween in 1968 and a member of what is now referred to as Generation X. The description of Generation X is not a bad one for me when I think about it. Taken from Wikipedia:

Members of Generation X, or Gen Xers, grew up in a time when there were more dual-income families, single-parent households, and children of divorce than when boomers were growing up. Consequently, many Gen Xers were latchkey kids, spending part of the day without adult supervision, as when they got home from school while their parents were still away at work. Gen Xers were the first generation to grow up with personal computers to some extent, thus becoming tech-savvy. They also experienced shaky economic times as children and young adults in the 1980s and '90s. Gen Xers are typically described as being resourceful, independent, and keen on maintaining work-life balance. They tend to be more liberal on social issues and more ethnically diverse than boomers.

This was pretty much my childhood. Both parents worked and we spent an awful lot of time on our own or with friends.

We did our homework if we wanted to or if we knew how. There wasn't much supervision in schoolwork, or anything, really. This was an important factor in our lives back then, because we learned quickly that at the end of the day, we were responsible for our own success or failure. We paid the consequences when we didn't put in the work.

I have a brother, Kevin, who is four years older than me and a sister, KathyAnn, three years older. I was the baby of the family. Whereas I was a Gen-X'er, they were at the tail end of the Baby Boomers. Despite our similar ages and identical family experience, we are different in so many ways. I was the one who got caught doing all the wrong things and constantly required a trip to the emergency room. I don't think I was accident prone. I'd say I was more "very-active" and perhaps a bit unlucky. My siblings had the occasional injury, whereas over the course of my childhood I had broken fingers, a collar bone, ankles, wrists and numerous cuts to my head and face requiring stitches. I suppose that qualifies as unlucky.

We were born in the United States in a Massachusetts town called Dedham, and in 1975, moved to Stoughton, another small Massachusetts town of about 25,000 residents. It took some time but I was very fortunate to have fallen in with a really good group of friends that were far more interested in riding bikes, playing sports and hanging out together than causing too much trouble. As an introvert, this suited me down to the ground.

Stoughton is approximately fifteen miles south of Boston so sports were a big part of my early years. With Boston being a great sports town with an amazingly rich sporting tradition, I was exposed to all four of the major sports in the USA at the time: baseball, football, basketball and ice hockey. Baseball and ice hockey attracted me the most, although, like many other kids, I tried all four as well as a few more just to see what they were like. I was always pretty athletic and in fairly good shape.

Back then, it was still unusual for the average family to go out to eat and most families had at least dinner together at the kitchen table with a home cooked meal consisting of relatively nutritious food. When we needed to go somewhere and it was within a few miles, we would usually take our bikes or just walk. Obesity certainly wasn't the norm as it is today. Generally speaking, life just required a little more energy in those days.

My father was an office manager for a trucking company and mother worked in accounts at an orphanage. They worked hard and earned themselves a respectable income to provide for my brother, sister and I. We didn't have everything, but we had what we needed and maybe a little more. At the age of four I fell in love with ice hockey and my father started me in an organised programme learning to skate by pushing around a milk crate. I still remember the old, heavy steel bladed skates on which so many of us little tikes first learned to stand up, with our ankles bent at 90-degree angles. The Boston Bruins had just won the Stanley Cup in 1972, beating the New York Rangers four games to two in a best of seven series. This, no doubt, was the catalyst for my interest in the game. I can't claim to be even remotely aware of their 1970 Stanley Cup victory. I can remember those nights when I was supposed to be in bed but snuck out to the living room and hid behind the couch to watch Bobby Orr, Derek Sanderson, Terry O'Reilly, and Gerry Cheevers play a hard-nosed game while my father sat on the couch having his beer and swearing at the old black and white TV. That was old time hockey and it was exciting. As a young kid, all I wanted was to grow up to be a professional hockey player.

In addition to ice hockey, I don't think I knew any boy my age who didn't play Little League baseball in our town and I was no different. There were some girls as well, so things had started to move in the right direction. In eastern Massachusetts, baseball was in our blood. The local population had a love/hate relationship with the Red Sox, who were a perennial disappointment in those days, having shown promise and sometimes coming close, but they hadn't won a World Series since 1918. We did have some remarkable talent with a young Carl Yastrzemski, Carlton Fisk, Jim Rice, Dwight Evans, Cecil Cooper, etc... I could write a book just on the local sports scene in Boston during the 70's and 80's.

There were also the legendary Boston Celtics basketball teams and a not yet well-established New England Patriots American Football franchise. The Celtics have a storied history and won a total of five championships in the 70's and 80's while the Patriots floundered during these years, for the most part, but did produce some pretty good talent along the way. They had a spark of excitement in the mid 80's under Raymond Berry, but they certainly weren't the team they would eventually develop into after 2001.

While there was no lack of sporting inspiration growing up, at that time, running, for me and nearly every other child, was considered more of a punishment. To be fair, I think that is probably why it took so long for the sport to make it to the mainstream population worldwide. Back then if you did something wrong in gym class you were forced to run laps. If you did something wrong in baseball you were forced to run laps. The same for nearly every activity there was. However, more recently it feels like nearly everyone has at least given the sport of running a try. I mean every one of every age, shape, and size which is amazing. Marathon running has exploded and the amount of people who can now call themselves a marathoner is a modern phenomenon. Additionally, nearly every town or village in the civilised world has a 5k or 10k event each year.

I went to a small, Catholic high school, Xaverian Brothers, in Westwood, Massachusetts between the years 1982 and 1986. It was, at the time, a school more known for academics than for sports but these days the sports world seems to have caught up. This is important for one reason in particular that is relevant to this story. Besides these being my formative years, I learned a tremendously valuable life lesson. A friend and I, who had played ice hockey for a number of years as youngsters, decided to try out for the freshman ice hockey team. We wanted to bring our passion for the sport to the next level. However, we both talked ourselves and each other out of going to the first tryout and that was it. I think deep down, neither one of us felt we were good enough and neither one of us ever played high school hockey. It is a decision I regretted back then and still do to this day. What I wouldn't give to go back to that day and take that uncomfortable first step. The decision as to whether we were good enough should have been in the coach's hands, not our own. That regret has taught me that if I say I want to do something then I am going to follow through. There is a great quote by Seth Godin that says, "The only thing worse than starting something and failing is not starting something." That says it all. I'll not say I've made all the right decisions since then or have not gambled and lost. I've made my share of mistakes and had some spectacular failures, but I've taken chances and have followed my heart.

After high school I went to university for a year, majoring in accounting, where I did next to no work and managed to lose my place. I had too much leeway around whether to attend class or not. *Not* won out a little too often. After that first-year failure, I had a decision to make. Instead of full time at school and part time work, I thought it best to turn those tables. I had been working in my local supermarket but an opportunity to work full time in the corporate office presented itself. I jumped at the chance and I was fortunate to have landed the position in the Consumer Information department. It was an interesting position, and I enjoyed the work, but more importantly, it opened up some doors that would have otherwise remained closed. This allowed me to study in the evenings and earn a decent living during the day.

In 1989 I earned my Associates degree in Business Management, which for me was an achievement in itself, but I'm not so sure what advantages it offered me. The supermarket experience was proving to have its own merit and I continued to advance from one position to another in that company.

This would be a trend throughout the course of my adult life. Drifting from one thing to the next without any clear focus on a destination. This is not necessarily a bad thing, it's just a fact. I had no clear idea of what I wanted to do for a career and no real prospects to build on. I was a drifter.

CHAPTER 3
EMERALD GREEN(ER) PASTURES

IN 1994, I was still working full time for that large regional supermarket chain in New England. At the time, the company was doing over $1 billion in sales and had around 120 stores scattered around all six New England states. I had moved my way up to Layout Coordinator, and was responsible for planning where the different categories of products went in the grocery, dairy and frozen food sections. The pay was good and I was moving up in the company. Things were generally positive. I also had a large circle of great friends and we did everything together. I still played recreational ice hockey and softball which were both enjoyable, but so was going to the pub afterwards where I enjoyed beer and cigarettes a little too much and a little too often. Still, despite being a smoker I was in fairly good shape back then, still lean and strong. Oh, and I was unattached.

Americans all believe we are a nationality in addition to being American. I considered myself Irish, that is until I met my future wife, Roisin, while she was visiting Boston. I was no more Irish at the time than I was German, Chinese or Scandinavian.

Us Americans are strange that way. A great many of us only call ourselves American when outside of the country. Roisin and I only spent a few days together but we really hit it off. I had taken her sightseeing, out to eat, and of course out to the pubs. When she flew back to Ireland, I was disappointed, but hey, things happen, right? About a week later she rang and we were both blubbering idiots on the phone. It was as if we had been long lost lovers who found each other after fifty years. I never thought I'd care about someone so much, especially after such a short amount of time together. I was wrong. I loved her accent, the different words she used, her unusual name, there were lots of little things to love.

After that first phone call, we started writing to each other and phoning every now and again. It was a real long-distance relationship, a little over 3,000 miles to be more accurate. As the cost to phone each other was around $1 per minute, the letter writing was far more economical. I would find myself writing to her several times a day. I was 26 years old and I was smitten. She consumed my thoughts and I couldn't wait to see her again. I'm sure my friends were sick of hearing about her and about Ireland.

This was way before the Internet was in every house and available at the flick of a switch. Mobile phones were becoming more popular, but there was nothing smart about them back then. They were for making phone calls, full stop. I was the typical *American*. I assumed Ireland was a little behind the times in every way. In my mind's eye everyone was a farmer and they still tilled the land with horses. I pictured the roads as dirt tracks. Black and white TV's and transistor radios formed the entertainment scene. These were some of the things my Irish grandfather would have talked about when I was younger. He had emigrated to America in 1936. It sounds crazy now, with the internet making the world so much smaller and readily accessible, that one would think like that, but that was how it was. It is embarrassing how we Americans think about the outside world. Little did I know there was a modern world beyond our borders.

I managed to visit Roisin in Ireland a couple of times, even just on long weekends. That's a very long journey in order to spend a couple of days. The first time I went was in the winter. At the time I don't think any of my friends or family had a passport. The thought of going anywhere outside the USA, or possibly Canada, was just something unheard of. But I knew I'd need one and applied for mine soon after Roisin first rang and we thought we might have something. I had literally just received my passport in the post and thought I'd take a trip over in November 1994. My bank account looked pretty healthy, so why not? I ended up catching a cold on the way over and on top of that, I'd never experienced jet-lag before. It's a strange thing, losing five hours of time. It hit me pretty hard but it was so good being together with Roisin and spending time with her in County Carlow where she was living and working as an assistant catering manager in a large factory.

I was lucky in that every time I visited Ireland, the weather was always decent. I was expecting rain, fog and clouds, like one reads about in books. What I got was usually some clouds but more blue sky than anything else. It was never really August-in-Boston hot, but Ireland is not exactly on the equator. It was as if Roisin placed a statue of the Child of Prague in the garden before each trip I made, which is an old Irish superstition for ensuring sunshine. She was doing everything in her limited powers to guarantee some glorious weather. Whatever she did seemed to do the trick.

She showed me all that Carlow had to offer, met some of her friends on a night out, visited Kilkenny Castle and enjoyed a day there exploring that charming medieval town, but all too soon it was time to go back to Boston. The flight home was terrible because my head was all stuffed up from my cold, so when we were descending into Boston's Logan airport my ears were going crazy and I was practically climbing the walls of the plane in agony. The pressure was relentless and my head felt like it would explode. I ended up with two ear infections and in quite a bit of pain for a few days after that, but it didn't put me off travelling.

We continued to write and phone each other and I went out again in the new year for another short visit, without any of the sickness drama from my previous trip. We made plans to tour the country in summer. As it happened, my next visit was in July of 1995. Roisin and I travelled all around Ireland during a spell of the nicest weather I've ever experienced here. We went to all the touristy spots like Blarney Castle in Cork, Killarney and Dingle in Kerry, Cliffs of Moher in Clare, Galway City, Sligo, Donegal, Derry, Belfast, Dublin. Everywhere we went was amazing and another truly excellent experience.

I did, however, have a wee surprise for Roisin. I had purchased an engagement ring before leaving Boston and kept it with me during our travels waiting for the perfect opportunity to present it. That night in Dingle felt like it was right. We had gone out for dinner, had a couple of drinks and went back to our B & B. I asked her to go for a walk with me along the beach. She refused, saying she was tired. I begged, she refused and suggested I go by myself. As she was completely oblivious to all the romance I was trying to create I finally gave up, got down on one knee and proposed, and it was accepted.

The pressure was off. After nearly a week of not wanting to leave the bag that had the ring in out of my sight, I could relax a bit. Looking back, Roisin says it was strange, at the time, that I seemed so nervous about my bags. But there you go, another major stepping stone towards what made me a runner. If I hadn't fallen in love with an Irish girl, I would have missed out on the person who introduced me to running. Would I have relocated out of the States where my life would have been monumentally different? Our lives are full of small, seemingly insignificant moments, that build up and lead us to those bigger life events and eventually to where we end up long-term. For me, my whole trajectory changed when Roisin made that phone call. That phone call was the first flutter of the butterfly's wings.

When I proposed, I also offered Roisin a deal. She would come out to live in Boston after we got married. If after five years she wanted to move back to Ireland, I would go. That was the deal and we both signed up to it. In December of 1995 she moved out to Massachusetts and for immigration purposes we got married by a Justice of the Peace in February 1996. In spring of that year, we started the house hunt. It took us to the small town of Foxborough, Massachusetts, only one mile from where the New England Patriots play their home games. It is a lovely town and not too far from my friends and family. We had found the perfect house for us to begin our new life together. It was old and full of character and we spent our first years together building a home. The big wedding took place later that year in August when we hosted a large contingent of Americans over in Fermanagh for the official church ceremony. This gang of Americans had a big surprise in store as none of them, myself included, had ever experienced an Irish wedding that goes on into the early hours of the morning.

The Americans, the Irish and everyone in between had a great time at the reception in County Monaghan. Roisin and I got to bed about 3am and were out the door again by 6am to catch our flight out of Dublin the next morning. We honeymooned in northern Italy for the first week in September 1996 where we had a blast before heading back to Foxborough to settle into our married life. In October we learned that Roisin was expecting our first child in June of the following year. The honeymoon was not only fun, it had been productive as well. Everything was moving faster than I ever imagined.

I was never very good around blood and needles or anything involving internal medicine. As a child, I would experience extreme nosebleeds and had to have my nose cauterised five times before I was 16. So one would think I could handle the sight of a bit of blood. Nope, not even close. This was evident when we went to birthing classes to get a better understanding of what was in front of us, and I nearly passed out during the discussions and demonstrations, at one point having to get up and leave the room. This was going to be an interesting experience.

When June of 1997 rolled around, I was in the birthing room for when our firstborn, Owen, arrived and I even managed to cut the umbilical cord. That part went fine, however, seeing the placenta out of the corner of my eye didn't do me any favours and my head went for a swim before I grabbed a seat and settled down. What would I be like if that was me having to get poked, prodded and probed? It wasn't worth thinking about.

Our daughter, Catraoine arrived hot on the heels of Owen, making her first appearance in October 1998. Roisin's experience with this second childbirth involved an epidural, which she didn't have with Owen. This, however, didn't really work as she was hoping. It caused more confusion than pain relief. At one point, she told the midwife she was having *transactions*. Evidently there was some overlap between childbirth and retail banking, her occupation at the time. In the end, Catraoine arrived with mother and daughter both safe and sound.

It was at this point that I had reached the end of my career hopes with the supermarket, as it felt like I was at the limit of advancement opportunities, and I began re-training in the field of IT. I had always been interested in computers and software, and had played around with it for a number of years, so it was a natural fit. At the end of 1999 I landed a new job as a Software Engineer at Seagreen Technologies, a small start-up software development house in Massachusetts. This change of direction offered a wider spectrum for growth and as a 32 year old, it was a good time to make the career change.

As the weeks and months got busier and more hectic with a new job and two small children, I had kept in the back of my mind that there was always the possibility of having to pick up sticks and move 3,000 miles east. My five-year deadline was quickly coming around and as the turn of the century approached, Roisin had a decision to make. Did she cherish her life in New England enough to raise her family there? Or did she want to move back to Ireland where she would be closer to her family and friends? To me the decision was easy. We had put down some roots and we both had good careers. We had four seasons of weather, each with its own attraction. We had a lovely home with family and friends close by. All four of us were in good health with a bright future ahead. Additionally, in March 2000 we found ourselves expecting once again, so if we were to relocate to Europe, we would be moving five of us.

Roisin didn't quite see things the same way. Her upbringing

was on a farm out in the County Fermanagh countryside. She loved the conveniences of living in our Massachusetts town and the high wages we were both earning, but there was a quality of life that only someone from outside the States could identify. Smaller schools, better healthcare and a much tighter sense of community were all pulling at her heartstrings. Not to mention you can take a girl out of Ireland, but you can't take Ireland out of a girl. She longed for a life closer to her large family, which consisted of her parents and seven siblings. It was her decision to make and after five years with two young kids and one on the way, Roisin was ready to move. I'll admit that it took me by complete surprise., I honestly thought that life in the States was everyone's dream. Her picture of an ideal home in Ireland was too strong and none of the bright lights in America were going to persuade her to stay and raise her family.

A YEAR TO REMEMBER

The year 2001 started out perfectly for our little family. We enjoyed the 2000 holiday season with friends and family and our third child was on the way. This one must not have fancied the cold Boston winter, and wanted to remain in the comfort of his mother's womb because he had been threatening to arrive early, but just kept holding off. In the afternoon before he was actually due, we took Owen and Catraoine to the cinema, at the start of a snowstorm, to see a holiday classic. About halfway through *The Grinch Who Stole Christmas*, Roisin went into labour and the fun began. We got the kids home and headed across town to the Brockton Hospital, where Aidan was born on January 21st. That morning, I had to dig my car out of a foot of snow in order to get home to the rest of the family, but we had another healthy boy and a positive start to the year.

We had just begun the second year of the new millennium, and it was also the time of the dot com crash. Just before the tech bubble burst in the US, investors were throwing money at any company involved with carrying out business on the internet. During my first year at Seagreen, the company was thriving and there was plenty of work. We were involved with a group of investors looking to develop an online presence and there was a relatively large pool of money promised for this work. The project was exciting because the work was cutting edge and the investment team included a world-renowned actor. The timing, however, was just a little off and as tech stocks started to drop in value, so did the amount of venture capital the team had promised for our project. As it turned out, the project never got off the ground and before long Seagreen Technologies, and a whole slew of other development companies, went out of business. I suddenly found myself out of work.

Every cloud has a silver lining, for this gave me the perfect opportunity to search for jobs in Ireland. It also coincided with what was called the Celtic Tiger, where the Irish economy was booming due to the technology industry. While tech companies were collapsing in the States, the industry was thriving in Ireland. On my first trip out to Dublin on the job hunt, I received two offers as a software engineer and I accepted one with AIG in Blackrock, Co. Dublin. The money wasn't close to what it would have been in the States, but trade-offs had to be made, and disposable income was one of them. Besides, I was moving for Roisin and the kids, not chasing a pot of gold for myself.

On May 3, 2001 our family flew together to Dublin, drove up to Fermanagh and awaited the delivery of the container with all our worldly belongings. I had two weeks before work started, and we took the time to get some of the basics in place. For these two weeks the sun shone like we were on the Costa del Sol, laying down the most unrealistic expectations in the history of mankind. We were both full of optimism for whatever the future held.

As I was to work in Dublin I rented a house in the town of Gorey in north County Wexford, the sunny southeast, and I commuted up to Blackrock every morning. Roisin and the kids moved into her brother Kevin's house up in Fermanagh while we searched for our permanent home. She certainly had her hands full with three young kids and me living three hours south. For the first four months, we lived apart during the week and only saw each other on the weekends. House prices in and around Dublin were astronomical, and neither of us wanted to live in the city, so we decided to expand our search radius. We looked up and down the country but nothing ticked all the boxes.

Roisin's parents soon came up with an idea to give us a plot of land up the hill and on the other side of the road from the family farmhouse. This wasn't what I had in mind. I had two conditions, and only two, for moving to Ireland. I wanted to live on the coast and I didn't want to live in the North. For the first condition, I've always loved the ocean, the peace that comes from listening to the waves roll onto the shore and the fresh sea air is fantastic for the soul. For the second condition, the peace process was still a little too fresh with the Troubles only officially coming to an end two years earlier with the signing of the Good Friday/Belfast Agreement. I may have been naive about that whole issue, but I knew 3,500 lives were lost over the previous 30 years. This was enough for me to want to live somewhere else in case peace didn't hold. Roisin was less concerned about coastal living, but had lived most of her life within the context of tension and divided communities so she too preferred to reside in the South.

The land proposal in County Fermanagh was interesting, though. It would set us up nicely and allow us to build a new house without financial pressures or any real time constraints. There was the small issue of the site location being 100 miles north of my work which would need to be addressed. I wrote a proposal to AIG requesting to work from home and commute to Blackrock every Friday morning. Unlike today's world, remote working was an entirely new concept for AIG and to be honest, back then, there wouldn't have been any companies in Ireland doing such a thing. But they took the leap of faith and allowed this to go ahead. On the 3rd of September, I logged in for the first time as a tele-worker. Only eight days later the world would change dramatically.

Just before 2pm on September 11th, my phone rang as I returned to my desk from lunch. It was one of the guys from the office. In typical Irish fashion, he calmly asked me if I was watching or listening to what was happening in New York. I replied that I wasn't and asked him what was going on. He just said I should hang up and turn on the TV. What I saw was coverage unfolding of the terrorist attacks in the United States. I was in a daze for a week, with my head glued to the television night and day. I took a few days off from work as the world tried to put together all that occurred on the day. This was a particularly difficult time for me as back then, I was a proud American at heart and here in Ireland I had absolutely nobody with whom to share this grief and anger; nobody who could see these events through the same lens. People would say they were sorry about what happened, but they understood why they occurred. To me, that made no sense. The people who were killed and injured were just ordinary people, Americans, no different from me. Good, hard-working people with families who loved them. I experienced profound loneliness and frustration over the course of the following months and struggled to explain to Owen when he asked why someone would do that.

Eventually, the world started turning again, myself included. The new remote work setup worked just fine despite the technological obstacles thrown up by living out in the country. We only had dial-up internet access and I was supporting an application for the company in five European countries, Finland, Germany, Italy, The Netherlands, and Poland. On the odd occasion I had to run scripts to insert up to half a million records into a database in one of these countries, over a dial-up VPN connection, which would literally take all night, but it always got done.

In the latter part of 2001, we began working with an architect to design our dream home where we could settle down and finally feel a sense of permanence. We managed to get the plans drawn up and approved so that over the course of 2002, construction of our new home began. We would occasionally visit the site to see the pieces coming together. Watching the site clearing, pouring the foundations, and the walls going up were all symbolic reminders of our fresh start, and we were full of hope and anticipation for the future. In October, Roisin and I got some more good news when we learned that we were expecting our fourth child.

THE UPS AND DOWNS OF GETTING SETTLED

Daniel made his welcome appearance in June, 2003 to complete our family. He was the only one of our four children to be born in Ireland, although all four have dual citizenship. He was such a contented baby, happy to sit and take in the world as his brothers and sister played around him. Our new house was just about ready, at least to the point where we could put on the finishing touches while living in it, so the six of us moved into our new place one week later, on Saturday, June 14. This was truly the beginning of the next chapter in my life. Everything was busy with four young kids and a new house that needed a lot of finish work, but I still managed to get out golfing with my father in-law and Roisin's brother-in-law every Sunday. It's too bad I wasn't getting any better at the sport. On the odd occasion, my brother-in-law Kevin and I would attempt to go out for a run, but we both found it way too hard. Even just a mile or two proved impossible. It didn't help that we live at the top of a big hill, but for some reason it wasn't just coming back up the hill that was tough; even going down made my lungs beg for forgiveness. I wouldn't figure out why it was this way for another seven years when I learned the concept of *pace*.

In the autumn of 2004, AIG made the decision to move our department's programming jobs overseas which once again left me out of work. I was, however, ready for a new challenge by this time anyway. I recognised a gap in the local market for IT products and services. There were no suppliers within 75 miles from my home. The only real option was online shopping, which wasn't as convenient or sophisticated as it would become. For the first time in my life, I decided to take sole responsibility for my own future and started a company in our local village building computers and offering hardware and software support. This was the start of many years of ups and downs as an entrepreneur.

I envisioned a few years of long hours and hard work, bringing my American customer service ideals to Fermanagh. My hope was that growth in the business would pay off quickly and give me the freedom to enjoy the fruits of my labour. It didn't take long for trade to gain traction but there were unexpected challenges. For one thing, I never ran a business before. There was a fine line between making a profit and taking a loss on every piece of work and in the first two years I barely broke even. For another thing, I found myself driving a van for hours each day and sitting behind a workbench repairing PCs. I was less active than ever and during this period, I could have taught a master class on how to pack on weight as I ploughed headlong into the worst shape of my life.

Golf was about the only sport I was taking part in during these years, which was at least something, but not particularly aerobic. My company wasn't going all that bad, but hadn't quite reached Fortune 500 status. My eating was out of control. I would go all day without eating a thing and when returning home at 8pm I'd be tired, hungry, and generally in a bad mood. I'd then consume everything within my reach. All I wanted to do was sit back and chill for a few hours but family life had different ideas. Roisin and I were always dropping off or picking up the kids at Gaelic football, Irish dancing, Ju-jitsu, or music classes. The stresses of life exacerbated my already impatient, intolerant and overall grumpy nature. My ill-tempered demeanour would see me snap at those I cared about most at the smallest irritations. I knew this wasn't fair, but I did nothing about it. I couldn't have been easy to live with. The weight-gain, the inactivity, and the pressure of running a business on a shoe-string budget combined to make me a heart attack waiting to happen.

This sedentary lifestyle and extra pounds soon led to me putting my back out. I had originally injured my back in 1996 when lifting a display in a supermarket. It was OK most of the time, but occasionally if I lifted something wrong, I would find myself in pain. In 2007, it became a real problem. It would seize up more and more often and when it did, it was completely debilitating. I couldn't walk, sit, stand or move without spasms shooting through my body for days at a time. This obviously caused problems in my work and duties at home. In addition, I had sore knees that not only interfered with work but also made playing with the kids uncomfortable.

In an attempt to ease some of the stress from work I started looking for some outside help in the form of potential business partners. This is when I made some very bad decisions as far as growing the company. I got into a business arrangement with a couple of partners who, although they appeared to be successful entrepreneurs in their own right, didn't help my cause. After a year in this new partnership, I found myself nearing bankruptcy and sitting on a mountain of personal debt. Needless to say, that was a very difficult time as my business went belly up. Looking back from afar, I count this as a very useful experience and I value it for teaching me a tough lesson. I recognised that nobody else could look out for me or my family as well as I could. In business, others would need to earn my trust, it would not be freely given.

I had to do something to make a living, so Roisin and I began a new company offering IT support once again, but this time it was back to just the two of us working out of the house. For every door that closes they say another door opens. Soon after starting up, I received a phone call, out of the blue, from someone looking for a business partner in Ireland to look after a big chunk of IT support work. The company who made contact had heard about me from some of the people I had done work for years before and I came highly recommended. This acted as a reminder that we should always endeavour to excel in everything we do, because sometimes the payback comes when you most need it. I was given two weeks to assemble a team of engineers to support a fleet of digital photo processing labs across the island of Ireland. This was a big break for us financially, and in 2009 our business offered us a bit of financial comfort for the first time since I left AIG. It did mean a lot more work for me and a lot more travelling the roads. With that came the continued unhealthy lifestyle and the big belly to match, and I fell further and further out of shape.

CHAPTER 4
OVERWEIGHT AND OUT OF SHAPE

IN FEBRUARY 2010, Roisin was invited to run a leg of the Belfast Marathon that April, as part of a five-member relay team. She had a five-mile section to run and her training got her out for a run two or three days a week. She would feel great after coming home, having finished a run. After a couple of weeks, she invited me to join her. I refused and came up with one excuse or another. It had been a while for me since my last attempt at running, which I hadn't enjoyed and found very difficult. Fitness wasn't my top priority, but eventually, seeing the benefits she was getting, I relented and headed out with her for a run or two where she did her best to drag me around.

We are very fortunate to have some great forestry roads up around us with beautiful scenery in County Fermanagh. There is one area called Jenkin Lakes that has a 2.3-mile loop and is a perfect location for someone to begin running without anyone seeing them. Therefore, it was perfect for me, who was self-conscious about being overweight, and had zero running style. I know better now, and think it is a myth that people will think you look funny when you're overweight and running. After all, who criticises someone out running and trying to improve their fitness, other than someone who wouldn't put the effort in themselves? All credit goes to those of us who try, as we all need to start somewhere. That said, at the time I definitely didn't want anyone seeing me.

My first few runs were just awful. I would get to a point about a quarter of a mile away from where I started and just stop. I couldn't go another step and my breathing was out of control. This continued for a few more of these terrible sessions, probably a half dozen attempts. Roisin was getting on far better than I was and this motivated me to keep trying. She found running useful in getting a break from the stresses of work and home life. I wanted to find that inner peace, even if only for a half hour at a time. I had to be missing something. Then one afternoon, on my own, it struck me like a bolt of lightning. What if I slowed down and ran *very* slow? Would that help? With that one small change, I managed to get beyond that quarter mile and for the first time complete the entire loop without stopping. I was brimming with pride and self-confidence. Roisin and I continued to run this loop together, keeping the pace in check, and before we knew it, we were challenging each other to do a second lap, then a third lap, and eventually a fourth. The day we ran four laps was an incredible experience for both of us. After so many bad runs and progress coming along so remarkably slowly, to put four full loops, over nine miles, behind us was awesome.

We completed a couple of races during these early days of running. First a 5k in August of 2010, and then a 10k in September. The running was still hard, though, so I felt like an imposter calling myself a proper runner. This is a ridiculous term, *proper runner*. If you run, you are a runner, but I think most runners start out with this feeling that they are not a real runner. There is a general perception that the really talented runners find it easy. However, the truth is that runners who have been participating in the sport for a while just understand that they will have to be uncomfortable for a while. I'm not sure anyone really enjoys the actual running, well not running hard anyway. But pushing through the pain and discomfort is where the magic happens.

During this time, the new business was coming along nicely. Financially, we were in the best place we had been in years. Life in Ireland was shaping up and starting to look good. Unfortunately, I was doing neither of those two things. A comfortable lifestyle isn't the best environment for one's physical well-being. Although I was running, I wasn't exactly leading the healthiest lifestyle. I was still overeating and over-drinking. The more the business grew, the less running I did. I was only getting out for the odd run these days, and once a week would be stretching the truth. I was tired from driving and working so many hours a day. I was attending IT support calls all over the country, making sure we hit all our targets. I'd have a trip to Cork on Monday, Achill Island on Tuesday, Belfast on Wednesday, there was always a call to attend somewhere. Success seems to always have its costs and for me it was my fitness. We had more disposable income and found ourselves eating out more and drinking a little more than before. The balance of success and fitness was tipping in the wrong direction when it could have easily levelled off with a little more focus.

I made the decision to hire another engineer and as the work team grew, the opportunity to travel and take the kids on holidays once again presented itself. On one occasion, returning from a summer holiday in Boston, I saw some photos of myself. I remember the moment I first saw these pictures and my jaw dropped. I had gotten severely overweight, without actually realising it. Going from a fairly skinny, athletic 30-year-old, weighing in at 10 stone 10 (150 lbs) to a 15 stone (215 lbs) 42-year-old. At 5'10" tall, 15 stone is much too heavy. As a matter of fact, it is considered obese on the NHS BMI calculator. I had a sore back, sore knees and little motivation. The photos shocked me. It was a slow road to obesity, and my lifestyle was clearly taking me in a dangerous and undesired direction. I made up my mind there and then that I was going to do something about it.

I was able to run up to the 10k distance, slowly, which is pretty damn good for anyone, but for an overweight middle-aged man it was a great starting point. What was lacking was a basic understanding of nutrition. Going out and running a 10k once or twice a week was never going to justify consuming buckets of junk food the rest of the week and sucking back a 12 pack of beer every weekend. Fortunately, there are some excellent resources out there on the internet. I found an app called MyFitnessPal, which turned out to be one of the most helpful software applications I had ever come across. There are loads more like it now, but this is the one I found and it completely transformed my eating habits.

Roisin didn't have much weight to lose, but most people would like to lose a few pounds. She set a goal to lose 10 pounds, probably more to help and support me on my mission than out of necessity. I, on the other hand, needed to drop thirty-five pounds at the very least. That would get me out of the over-weight category. My brother, sister-in-law, and sister also got involved and we all tracked our food intake together on the app and kept each other accountable. I logged everything I consumed. Learning how many calories your individual body uses in order to lose, gain and maintain weight is a very useful exercise. We are all a bit different, but there are some very useful guidelines to help get started. I began by setting a daily goal of 1,600 calories. What I found was that the app gave back calories for doing exercise. For example, if I did an hour of cardio my calorie goal increased by 350. However, this didn't seem to add up on the scale. I found it far more useful for weight-loss to forget the calories burned and stick to my daily goal of 1,600. This was enough to keep me eating sufficient quantities of healthy food and lose weight at the same time.

Up until this point, I had no real understanding of how much I was eating. It just never occurred to me. I also thought I had a general sense of nutritious food and junk food, but to be honest, it wasn't correct. Big corporations have the marketing budget to push their messaging, making one believe they are choosing healthy options, when in fact nothing could be further from the truth. Logging my daily intake ensured I made better choices. I learned quickly that water was my friend, and that if I didn't waste my calories on drinks, I could eat more food and enjoy my food more. Prior to this time, the only water I drank was in my coffee, which I would drink all day, or in the beer I consumed. After starting this new regime, I made a point to drink at least two litres of water per day. If I was going to have any beer, I made sure to log it and take it into my daily calorie calculation. It took some getting used to, but I was making the adjustments.

The pounds started coming off quickly and we were all enjoying the journey. Roisin and I were running more often, and on the days we weren't running we were using the stationary bike, the cross trainer, doing a circuit, or some weight training at the house. We were both motivated. By August of 2012, I got down below the 200 lb mark for the first time in years. In September I got under 190 and by the middle of October, I was under 180. I had hit the initial goal of losing 35 pounds, but I wasn't ready to stop this weight-loss train. Roisin had also lost more than she set out to lose and was maintaining below her goal weight. For me, I found the challenge and the discipline enjoyable. It was a sense of achievement.

I was learning so many valuable lessons. When you know what you are eating, you can make the necessary adjustments and better choices required to hit specific goals. I learned the importance of each of the macronutrients and how to make the best use of protein, carbs and fats. Carbs being used to fuel a workout and a balanced mix of all three to promote muscle growth and recovery after a workout. Weight loss was much easier with the support of friends and loved ones, particularly Roisin, who I shared meals with. For us, losing weight was about a lifestyle change, not the latest fad diet, eating trends or short-term meal replacements. There are so many healthy options that taste amazing, including foods I'd never heard of or considered eating. Foods like oily fish, ground turkey, and quinoa were great choices. We planned every meal and prepared them from scratch. Planning meant we weren't caught out being hungry and reaching for the quick and easy bad choice. I loved food even more, now that I had an appreciation for the nutritional impact of the ingredients, but I balanced everything out and never deprived myself of the foods I wanted. Yes, I would still go out to eat, have the odd takeaway, and even occasionally over-indulge on junk. The difference was that I was aware of it and lived by the rule of eating well *most of the time* and didn't get anxious about what I ate *some of the time*. I had a strategy for losing weight and knew I could do it.

In November 2012 the bathroom scale read just under 170, which meant I had lost forty-five pounds in a little over a year. I felt great and had replaced some unhealthy habits with new ones that were much healthier. At this point I was exercising regularly and running more often. Running was starting to feel more enjoyable, although, as Greg Lamond says, "It never gets easier, you just get faster."

CHAPTER 5
WOW, I LIKE THIS RUNNING MALARKEY

I HAD GROWN to enjoy running as a weight-loss tool. I have always been somewhat of a data nerd and this was obvious with my use of the food tracking application. I enjoyed entering all of my information in and reviewing the data on a regular basis. Running lends itself to this type of analysis. There is something incredibly satisfying about seeing improvement; in pushing yourself to your limit and sitting back to take stock of how far you've come. I loved those really challenging runs where after arriving back home, I'd hardly be able to lift my legs out of the car or walk into the house without looking like Frankenstein's monster. The pain was the investment in my growth. I was making weekly deposits into my *health account* and someday I may need to call on these miles, these sacrifices, this pain, and make a withdrawal. As for growth and improvement, what better way to track progress than by taking part in the sport's ultimate challenge, racing.

It's true that most people aren't racing against their fellow competitors, but against themselves and who they were yesterday. Unless you are among the lucky few who can genuinely compete against the best of the best, even locally, it isn't about winning. For most of us, improvement is the best motivating factor in the sport. I had started my lifestyle change when I came to grips with food and nutrition to improve my health and well-being. I had no real interest in racing, but I thought it was worth trying so I could lay down a benchmark to gauge where I was and see if I could get better. Running is hard, racing is harder, but the benefits are among the most transformational I ever experienced.

Racing, it turns out, is not just about skill, but also a test of character, and it takes both to be really good at it. I ran my first 5k race in Clones, as hard as I could, without stopping. There was a battle going on, between my head and my heart, the entire way around the course. My head was telling me I had to stop, and my heart was telling me, "No way are you going to stop!" I was able to face the discomfort and continue until I reached the finish line. I believe that is what makes runners a breed apart from the general population. We have that internal fire burning so hot that when our brain tells us it's too hard, we give our brain the finger and carry on.

Running is very much like life. Both are hard and sometimes unfair. Both can be thrilling and heart-breaking. Running has also helped me find the alone time I require. Making it possible to separate from the hustle and bustle and be in my own space, just me and the road or me with nature. We've all had those days when we require solitude to work through a difficult problem or come to grips with a personal dilemma. Those hours on the road putting one foot in front of the other, the wonderful monotony, the rhythmic, mesmerising cadence maintaining a clear head for the duration of a run...it is therapy disguised as exercise. I always feel lighter of heart and mind after returning from a run. The more I ran and the more I raced, the more I improved, the more I enjoyed it.

The following pages describe some of the first races I took part in and the impact they had on me, because they all impressed something upon me. Each of these early races left an unforgettable memory, toughened me up, and brought me together with other runners. I learned so many lessons about running and about myself as an individual. For the first time in my life, I searched my inner self and found a strength I didn't know I had. I was privileged to meet some truly inspiring, passionate people who, to this day, I call friends. Each of these early races provided the next building block in my life, taking me from an overweight IT engineer to a passionate runner pursuing a healthy life.

I followed the natural progression, from a casual runner to taking part in a 5k. From the 5k I went to the 10k, then to the half marathon, and on to the marathon. I don't know why, but for so many runners the marathon is the holy grail of distances. At the time it seemed completely beyond my grasp, but then again so did the 10k before I did one. Everything is impossible, until it isn't. Looking back, I can see that taking the smaller steps up in distance made the entire process more enjoyable and at each stage the self-belief and confidence grew. I doubt it would have been the case if I jumped in at the half marathon distance and struggled. I may not have continued in the sport. Thankfully, I took the path I did.

WAS THAT A 10K OR A VIOLATION OF HUMAN RIGHTS

I completed the Clones 5k in August 2010, so the next logical step was to move up to the 10k distance. Again, Roisin and I continued to run during the week and had actually managed to build up to about eight miles in training, so we knew we could manage the 6.2-mile distance without stopping. On September 25, 2010, there was another race close by in a townland called the Knocks. They called this race "The Climb." At least they weren't trying to hide the fact that this was going to be a challenge. The 10k went out a country road a little under 1k before turning right. This right turn took us downhill for about 3k. This was quite the descent, being quite sharp in places, making it a technical downhill stretch. All I knew was that I had to move my legs quickly in order to avoid falling and rolling the entire length of the steep decline. This made the thought of the return trip back up all the more ominous. At the bottom, we turned right for about 1k before making another right-hand turn where we started "The Climb." This next 4.5k was the toughest experience I had to date while running. Straight uphill, and even when the road appeared to level off ahead, it just became another bend that continued to climb up and up. My pace was only slightly faster than walking, and I wasn't the only one as there were plenty of walkers around me who just couldn't face this hill. It was truly horrible and my brain fought me with every stride. It didn't seem possible to get enough oxygen into my lungs to take another step. Eventually, I reached the crest of the hill and there was only about 500m to go over a flatter, but still undulating, section of the road.

Crossing that finish line in a time of 58:40 was pure elation. Roisin and I ran the entire course together, encouraging each other, and we finished side by side. Similar to my experience in Clones, there was very little enjoyment in the racing itself, but the sense of joy when it was all said and done was the real payoff. As the heart rate comes down, breathing becomes easier and the runner's high hits. That's when it becomes worth it and incomparable to any other activity I've taken part in.

The first 5k and 10k were the best experiences I could have asked for. When the little voice told me to stop, I thought to myself, "What would happen if I don't stop?" The answer wasn't that I'd collapse or that I'd die, but simply that I would just keep going. It would be slow, but it would be another step towards the finish line. All progress is good progress.

After finishing the tough 10k, the hospitality at the Knocks Community Centre made amends for what they put us through. I got a taste for the camaraderie of runners as we sat around chatting, recovering, and enjoying the fantastic spread of food the organisers and volunteers had out. We all had the shared experience of running an extremely difficult race. Some managed to complete it in half the time as others, but it was a level playing field as far as effort. We could all respect each other for completing it. Whether young or old, those well off or not so well off, the skinny and not so skinny, the seasoned runners and the newbies, the fast runners and the slow, it just didn't matter. We were all runners and we all finished the race.

THAT'S A LONG WAY TO GO

There is a fairly popular half marathon in the Tyrone County town of Omagh that takes place annually in the spring. Having competed in our first 10k in September, we set our eyes on our first half marathon for April 2, 2011. Omagh is only about 20 miles away, so we drove the twisty road over Fintona mountain to the event, picked up our numbers and pinned them on our running tops with far more confidence than in previous races. This was a big field with over 1100 participants. Big for us anyway, considering our race experience consisted of only two other events that drew mostly locals. I was excited to be there. I could tell by the butterflies fluttering in my stomach as we lined up, awaiting the starter to release the runners onto the town. We didn't really know many other runners at this time, so the mass of people on the start line was a little intimidating, but we ignored the unfamiliarity and found ourselves in the middle of the pack.

It started without a hitch, but I'd never been in such a large bunch of runners before, so it felt strange to be jogging so slow at the start as the field advanced shoulder to shoulder. Things started to spread out by the time we took the first left turn onto the main road heading up the town centre. It's not a particularly scenic course, but it draws a big field of runners of all abilities. It falls early in the racing season and fits nicely into the schedule for those preparing for the Belfast Marathon. The route heads toward the rural areas of town and traverses some hills. On and on, up and down, this course challenged my stamina and had me questioning if I was ready to take on such a distance.

Eventually, a little over two hours after the start, the course began to descend back towards the town centre and the leisure centre where the finish line beckoned. I took the final left-hand turn, then reached the running track for the final 400 metres. Overjoyed, I crossed the line with a time of 2:04:38. Roisin was just a few minutes behind me at 2:08:01. When we saw each other, we both felt a flood of relief that we had completed our first 13.1-mile race. Soon, relief turned to joy as our hearts filled with pride. Despite the muscle aches, we smiled for the remainder of the day.

There was, however, one tragic occurrence on that day. A young 25-year-old police officer, Ronan Kerr, was killed when a car bomb went off as he drove away from his home in Omagh at 4pm. The police believe the bomb was in place at the time that all the runners passed by the parked car earlier in the day, as the course ran past it. That served as a reminder of how tenuous times were, even twelve years after the signing of the Northern Ireland peace agreement.

AN EVEN LONGER WAY TO GO

A year went by without any racing and very little running while my business continued to gain momentum. Work was going so well by the middle of 2012 that we decided we could afford to hire another engineer to cover the remaining calls I was handling. This allowed me to place a greater focus on fitness, which had become more important in my life. My weight loss journey reached a high point when I added strength training, cardio, and running back into my routine. By this time, my back and knee pain were a thing of the past. Obviously, they had been caused by the extra weight I had been carrying. This was a time to really challenge myself and I lifted my gaze to the marathon. Why not? By November of 2012, I had dropped 40lbs, which is 2 stone 12 pounds in old money, and I was still going in the right direction.

Roisin and I signed up for the Belfast Marathon, to take place on May 6, 2013. Our whole story had evolved from a weight-loss endeavour to a passion for running. We were both experiencing so much enjoyment, satisfaction and pride in our running that the physical fitness was just a massive bonus. I had a newfound self confidence that I wanted to cash in on while it was still fresh.

Come January, our training began in earnest. We didn't have a strict plan, other than trying to go that little bit further each week. We still had no formal coaching or any other running friends nearby so our only goal was to finish the entire 26.2 miles without stopping. My sister-in-law from Boston, Ann Marie, had run a marathon before, and she offered helpful advice such as, "Only increase your distance a little each week," and told us to take nutrition in the form of gels along the way. She was quite positive in her encouragement which we both found hugely beneficial.

I recall quite clearly those weekend long runs where we would either be up at our local forestry or along the flattest roads we could find to complete our run, hobble back to the car, drive a short distance home and not be able to get out. As the long run distance crept up and up each week so did the amount of post-run recovery time required. I still feel bad for our non-running friends forced to listen to us talk about our training. It had totally taken over our lives. We must have been the most tiresome and boring company. Hopefully, this is no longer the case, but I dare to say things may not have changed all that much. It's just that our company tends to be other runners now.

Nutrition was of the utmost importance. As I was doing more and more miles, I was eating more and more calories than I had been over the past year. It felt strange, but it felt great. I'm a big fan of food. I can count on one hand the things I won't eat, so as the calories increased so did my happiness. We had to fuel those fifty-mile weeks with something. The key was the quality of the food we consumed, and it put our dietary knowledge from the previous year and a half to the test. Many new marathon runners find they gain weight when training. It isn't a licence to eat all the food, but more, good food. After a long run, we came home and ate a good recovery meal, which we would have prepared before going out. Refuelling in this way ensured that we got the best results from our training without putting on any pounds.

During this time, we were also looking after our successful technical managed services company, which meant our focus was split between running a business covering the entire island of Ireland and running the roads and trails around County Fermanagh. We were going well on both counts. Our four kids were getting on well in school, but they too were probably sick to their stomachs listening to us talk about running. However, we believed if we were eating right and exercising, it could only be providing a positive influence for them. On the first of January 2013, Owen was 15, Catraoine 14, Aidan about to turn 12, and Daniel was 9. They weren't overly keen on some of the dinners we were preparing, but hey, eating healthy isn't a crime. We were all relatively happy and healthy.

At this point, I should add that we didn't have any running gadgets like a GPS watch or anything. I did have a running app, Runtastic, on my phone, but it was a bit of a hassle to strap my phone onto my arm or hold it in my hand, so I didn't always use it. I'm a tech guy, so I do like to analyse things. I have since had a number of different running watches, and I'd be lost without them. Not so much during the run, but for the post mortem analysis when I get back. Like many say these days, if it's not on Garmin or Strava, it didn't happen.

By the end of January, my training was progressing well for the May Belfast Marathon. So much so that come the middle of

February, I felt I could handle the distance and on Monday the 18th of February, I started looking for a marathon I could do in the upcoming weeks instead of waiting until May. As luck would have it, the Marathon Club Ireland group were putting on a race that Saturday, February 23rd. I got hold of the organiser to see if I could enter and he assured me that it would be no problem. It was in a small town in County Clare called Sixmilebridge, about 175 miles south of Fermanagh. I booked a hotel room and went down after work on Friday night. Roisin's training was going well too, but it was still a little early for her to tackle the distance with confidence, so I was on my own. Talk about a fish out of water. This group was mostly made up of members of the 100 Marathon Club Ireland, which is a club for people who have completed or attempting to complete at least 100 marathons.

At the start line, among all these experienced marathoners, the organiser called me out as a first timer and I got a warm round of applause and a "Welcome to the club" greeting from everyone. My intention was to try to stick to a 10-minute mile pace. I had no watch, no phone or anything, so it was going to have to be determined by how I was feeling. The ultimate goal was to finish the entire 26.2 miles, non-stop. Standing on the start line on that February morning, I was a bundle of nerves. I had so many doubts about what was going to happen. The weather was cold, dry, and cloudy, but not freezing and not windy. It was to be good conditions for a long run.

One of the great things about marathons is that there is time to have a few words of a chat with people, especially if they aren't too concerned about racing for a time. I fell in with different people along the way who offered their advice, support and most importantly inspiration. This was a far cry from the shorter races when it was a struggle to breathe. I found this more comfortable and more in-line with my training runs.

Mile after long mile ticked by. Every step was one step closer to the finish. I clearly remember the uphills and the downhills and how extremely far it always felt until I would reach the finish line. There is something comforting to me about a long run. Particularly when the weather is agreeable, I spend the long miles pondering life and imagining the feeling of getting to the end; visualising the coffee and cake when it's all over. I eventually crossed the finish line, to the appreciation and applause of quite a few other runners who would have been thinking back to their first marathon. The finish time was 4:22:58 which is almost exactly a 10-minute mile. As a first timer, I was just over the moon. I finished and, most importantly, I knew now that I could run 26.2 miles without stopping. Going forward, I could now call myself a marathon runner, which had a lovely ring to it.

Sixmilebridge was an overwhelmingly positive experience and one I will always be grateful for. This was also such an unusual thing for me to do. I went well beyond my comfort zone to make contact with someone I didn't know about running a race 175 miles from home, and on my own no less. It sounds like nothing now, but back then, that was an extraordinary situation for me to put myself in.

Something in me was changing for the better. There was a self-confidence building. It was showing in my actions and in my appearance. Clothes were fitting me better, and as a matter of fact, I needed an entirely new wardrobe. I still have some of the shirts I used to wear and they are now like dressing gowns on me. My old jeans with a 38-inch waist can now fit two of me.

Roisin was delighted with my success in the marathon and

we both took encouragement from my experience. I had a little more experience now and had picked up tips and advice from more seasoned runners, which I shared with Roisin. It was just what we both needed. We felt ready, or at least as ready as one can feel going into our first fairly large, city marathon.

TRAGEDY VISITS BOSTON

April 15, 2013 is a day that will go down in running history as an utter tragedy. A display of the absolute worst of humanity. Ironically, despite the terrorist's intentions, what was also demonstrated during the event and ever since was the sheer brilliance of humanity. The grit and determination of the people of Boston and the remarkable camaraderie of the running community as well as the greater sporting world were also on display. It was a stressful and concerning day for every Bostonian, but I had a personal interest as my brother Kevin and his wife, Ann Marie, were running this race.

At 14:49 that fateful Monday afternoon, the world of marathon running changed. The first of two pressure cooker bombs went off near the finish line on the famous Boylston Street. Only fourteen seconds later a second similar device went off just yards away. We should never forget the names of the three people senselessly killed that day. 29-year-old Krystle Marie Campbell from Medford, MA was killed by the first bomb. 23-year-old Lü Lingzi from Shenyang, Liaoningand, China, and young eight year old Martin Richard from Dorchester, MA were both killed by the second bomb. The innocence of the three victims really stands out. They were just there to absorb the inspirational atmosphere that only the finish line at the Boston Marathon can provide. The most heart-breaking image, the one that really touched me was the image of Martin, that came out in the days following the incident, where he is holding his now famous sign he made in 2012 saying, "No more hurting people. Peace." That message is as poignant as it gets.

We should also not forget the more than 260 injured, including 17 who lost limbs. This was a violent, purposeful act and it still hurts to think about it. This event is always a family friendly event full of inspiration and hope, and that came crashing down in an instant. At the time, four hours, nine minutes and forty-three seconds after the start of the third wave of runners, there were still over 5,700 runners who hadn't completed the course. Boylston Street was streaming with runners approaching the finish line, many completing their first marathon, which in normal circumstances would be a life changing experience. For others, this may not be their first, but Boston is always special. Instead, they got a life-changing experience that they had never asked for.

There is one more name that many people might recognise: Mr. Bill Iffrig. Bill, at the time, a 78-year-old avid runner competing in his third Boston Marathon was the closest runner to the first bomb when it went off. He can be seen getting knocked off his feet and stumbling down. He stayed down for a moment or two, but someone helped him up and, in a determined *runner's spirit* sort of way, completed the final 20 yards to the finish line. He completed the race in an official time of 4:03:47. It is hard to know what goes through someone's thoughts at a time like that, but for Bill there was an instinct to just get over the line and finish the race. He had a never give up attitude and that was on display throughout the day in that city.

I was following Kevin and Ann Marie using the marathon tracker app, but I stopped briefly to drive my boys to Ju-jitsu class. While there, I got a text message asking if I heard about the marathon and that something bad had happened at the finish line. I immediately got on the phone and checked out what was going on. It would have been 7:49 pm in Ireland when the bombs went off, and so this must have been a little after 8 pm when I was notified. I phoned my parents to check if they had heard from Kevin or Ann Marie, but nobody had heard anything from them. It was actually about an hour later that we got news that they were OK. What a relief.

They had reached somewhere around mile 23 when police moved the runners off the road to allow for emergency vehicles to pass. At this point nobody who was still on the course knew what was going on. It was obvious that there was an issue, though, as the number of ambulances, fire engines and police cars speeding past increased. Kevin and Ann Marie managed to make it to mile 25, where the course was officially closed, and they were told to stop. They had their phones with them and when they switched them on to check what was happening, notifications started pinging away. Friends and family were contacting them to see if they were alright. It was an hour or so from the time of the bombings that they contacted us, and the word spread quickly through the family. Fortunately, Kevin had also brought his bank card, because soon after they stopped running, the chilly April weather started to set in. They obviously couldn't get to their kit bags from the bag drop. As they wandered the city trying to figure out their next move, a runner who had already finished the race gave Ann Marie her finisher's foil blanket and told her that she needed it more than her at the minute. The kindness of strangers was starting and the generosity of the people of Boston was already on display. They found a TJ Maxx just before it closed for the day and were kindly given a few minutes to get in and pick out some warm clothes as businesses throughout the city closed down. Meanwhile the mobile networks in the city were shut down for security reasons and we didn't hear too much from them until later that night.

The images from that day, in the middle of all the chaos and confusion, show otherwise ordinary individuals performing extraordinary acts of courage and kindness. I am moved every time I see the images of Carlos Arredondo running alongside Jeff Baumann after helping him into the wheelchair; and Matt Smith, the man in the red t-shirt, comforting Sydney Corcoran on the ground; all of the runners and spectators helping each other. Despite the divisions in the world, there are so many stories from this day, from small gestures to acts of extreme courage, that prove humanity still has so much in common. This event solidified the running world and our commitment to ourselves, our sport, and each other. Death and destruction was delivered to unsuspecting victims for the second time in my three years of running. It's hard to see how anything other than pain and suffering was accomplished by these incidents.

So, the big question is, how is this relevant? Well, because they didn't get to finish Boston, Roisin and I asked Ann Marie and Kevin to join us and run in Belfast. They decided they would, and that laid the groundwork for a truly wonderful experience of running a marathon in tribute to the victims, survivors and all the people involved in the Boston Marathon. It was also what we thought of as a once in a lifetime experience: running a marathon together as a family.

THE BELFAST CONNECTION

On May 6, 2013, Roisin and I were as prepared as we were going to be. We had all the miles in the bank, I had done my test run in Sixmilebridge, and we had new motivation after the Boston bombings. Kevin and Ann Marie were ready to complete this challenge as well. It would be the first marathon for both Roisin and Kevin while Ann Marie and I would be looking to complete our second. We were all excited and a little nervous. The plan was that we were going to stick together the whole way around, come hell or high water.

There was quite a buzz at Belfast City Hall for the beginning of the marathon with runners, spectators and media milling about. In total, there were a little over 17,000 participants in the event. Most of these were members of relay teams, but there were still around 7,000 runners on the start line when the organisers of the event held a moment of silence in memory of the lives lost in Boston. It touched the four of us personally. Kevin and Ann Marie had brought the four of us running t-shirts with "Boston Strong April 15, 2013" printed on them. We wore these and it gave each of us a sense of pride that we were running for all those involved with the tragedy.

Waiting on the start line for the gun to go off I was full of excitement as opposed to nerves. It took a couple of miles for us to get into a rhythm, but we did, and the first few miles were quite enjoyable with those around us still positive and full of optimism. We were towards the back with other runners of roughly the same ability and similar goals. We had some chat with other runners, but were enjoying being together as a foursome.

As is true with most city marathons, the supporters were out in big numbers, sharing sweets or oranges or just shouting encouragement, making the entire experience such a joy. If one can call hours of pain joy. There were times when some of us were feeling stronger than the others and it changed throughout the morning. The noise on some sections of the course was pretty amazing, and it was a real eye-opening experience for Roisin and I both, who had never been involved in a truly big running event yet. Belfast is a unique city for many reasons considering its history. Its most famous claim to fame being that the Titanic was built in the Harland and Wolff shipyard back in 1912. Today, the two giant cranes, Samson and Goliath, dominate the skyline at the docks. Belfast is also famous for the hundreds of murals painted on buildings and walls throughout the city, each telling a story from the past. Additionally, the Peace Walls, which divide the city into Catholic and Protestant areas, have become quite an attraction. This course gave the runners a view of each of these landmarks. For my brother and Ann Marie, one of the many things they noticed while running through the peace walls was that the lamp posts changed from having Irish flags to having Union Jacks or the Ulster flag flying from them.

People were proud of their local neighbourhoods and they came out to show their support to the runners. We saw some signs and tributes to the Boston Marathon along the way, including a stand from the Belfast Fire Brigade, which were all touching and very much appreciated by us Bostonians.

Ultimately, we were all still inexperienced runners and had a lot to learn. As we went along, the day warmed up and Kevin began to overheat somewhat. Dehydration began taking its toll at around mile 16. Although Kevin and I were holding a steady pace just ahead of our partners for the first 15 miles, it was here that he started to slow down and we dropped behind while Ann Marie and Roisin pushed just ahead. Then Kevin ran into some difficulty. This was the definition of *hitting the wall*. It just so happened to hit him a little earlier than anyone could have expected and our pace slowed to a crawl. We trudged along the course, walking the odd stretch, and then jogging again when he found it possible. It was somewhere around mile 23 that we passed by the finish line where we could see the crowds and hear the announcer calling all the runners in by name. The only problem is that it's on the wrong side of the Lagan River. We still had over three miles to go. Ugh!

We had the long climb up the Ormeau Road, which under normal circumstances would be considered just a gradual pull, but getting towards the end of a marathon, and particularly for Kevin, after crashing into the dreaded wall so hard, this wee pull was more of a torture. There was never any question that we were going to finish this together, so when we hit the down-hill stretch back to Ormeau Park we took our time, encouraged Kevin and eventually hit the gates leading to the last 50 metres to the finish line. It was here that Roisin suggested we link arms and cross over the timing mat together in a time of 5:15:29 as the announcer called us out over the tannoy. There are some wonderful photographs that Roisin's brother-in-law, Sean, took of that moment with the four of us wearing our Boston Strong t-shirts and smiling ear to ear. He snapped quite a few treasured photos on the day, from the start to the finish, capturing what was a truly momentous achievement for us. We have so many great memories from this event and will never forget the spirit in which we all stuck together to carry each other over the finish line.

We got our bottle of water and a bag of Tayto Crisps at the

finish and we found a spot to sit down on the grass in the park. Kevin was ready for something more substantial and got a burger from the chip van, and he was fresh as a daisy. How he managed to feel so good after getting a short rest and some water I'll never know. I could barely sit down as my body had seized up, and I told the others they could forget about getting me back up any time soon. The rest of us had a coffee, recovered for about thirty minutes and had some laughs with Sean. Before long, we started back to the bus, which took us to the city centre and our hotel. Now is probably a good time to mention that one should not rehydrate, post marathon, with Guinness and Jameson and both Kevin and I learned this lesson the hard way! Still, big city marathon number one done and in the books. Best of all Kevin and Ann Marie were able to get the benefit of the training put in for Boston.

THIRD TIME LUCKY

Belfast lit the marathon fuse for Roisin and I. We loved the experience and were confident that we could better our time from our first big marathon. We hit the internet searching for the next one we could take on while we were in decent marathon shape. The Cork City Marathon, scheduled for the Monday bank holiday, June 3rd, seemed to hit all the right notes. The only issue was that it was a four-and-a-half-hour drive down. Although we could stay the night before, we would have a very long drive home immediately following the race. On Sunday, June 2nd we travelled the 220 miles to Cork City and spent the night at the sponsoring hotel. This time it was just the two of us and we were each going to run our own race and see how fast we could do it. I was brimming with confidence, maybe too much so, but still, I had convinced myself that I could do better than the 4:22 I ran in Sixmilebridge. Roisin was also full of positivity, knowing that she could better our 5:15 in Belfast, so we were in it for PB's.

Along the way I bumped into a number of the runners from the Sixmilebridge race and got into a conversation or two. These runners from the Marathon Club Ireland don't miss a chance to run a marathon so they were all here, and I enjoyed the craic.

It was a very nice warm day, which was great for me as, unlike most Irish runners, I'm a warm weather enthusiast. The course was interesting and I got to see a lot of the city. One of the more unique experiences was running through the Jack Lynch Tunnel and hearing the runners ahead shouting the "Oggy, Oggy, Oggy" chant and getting the response "Oi, Oi, Oi," with voices echoing loudly. I've now experienced that in most of the races in Ireland, but that cracked me up at the time.

Overall, the race was terrific. The course and the support were brilliant. The one thing that I didn't expect was that when we hit the halfway point, or thereabouts, the half marathon race merged with the full marathon. All the space we fought for during the first half had to be regained at the midway point when another wave of runners crowded the streets and all momentum was lost. A novice like me found it difficult to cope with at the time, but I suppose in the whole scheme of things this was a small detail I would need to get used to in races.

After another gruelling race of 26.2 miles, we both recorded personal bests, and I crossed the finish line with my first sub four-hour milestone in the bag with a time of 3:57:40. Roisin finished in 4:17:44. What a feeling for both of us. This was the first time I set myself a personal time goal, in this case doing better than Sixmilebridge, where I laid down the marker.

We did leave it all out there and we were both spent at the

finish. Unfortunately, we had a two mile walk to get to the bag drop and then back to the hotel. Not to mention a very long drive ahead of us. I looked rather like the tin-man from the Wizard of Oz and it's so funny because that is exactly how all the TV commercials portray the condition of runners post-marathon. We eventually managed to get back to the hotel where we showered, checked out, and loaded up the car. Our trip back home took us across the last mile of the marathon course. One of the more unforgettable scenes for me was when we saw one individual still on the course. She had about a mile or so to go and it would have been over the six-hour mark into the run. To me, this was inspirational. That effort was far more impressive than most of us on the course on that day. Here was someone who decided to take on the challenge, decided she wasn't going to give up, and persevered and finished a massive accomplishment.

CHAPTER 6
STRENGTH IN NUMBERS

FULLY ADDICTED TO RUNNING NOW, a friend convinced me to go to a training session with the local club in Enniskillen. I was nervous, as I think anyone would have been. I went anyway, feeling in my heart that I didn't belong there and not knowing at all what to expect. I may have run a few races including three marathons, but I had never trained on a track or in a group with experienced runners. In addition, I saw what real runners looked like when I did go to those races. Those men and women at the front of the start line, wearing their club vests, with the latest running gear. I saw the times they were posting at the finish. I was not in their league at all.

For my part, I'll say this was the best decision I was ever coerced into taking. Up until now, I still had very few friends on this side of the Atlantic. Very few people that would have considered me a friend anyway. I had struggled for years with loneliness and a pinch of low self-esteem since moving to Ireland, and especially after putting on a whole lot of weight.

Joining the club meant that things changed dramatically and rather quickly after this fateful day.

It was June of 2013, just a week after the Cork Marathon and I hesitantly dragged myself down to the track and took the all important first step out of the car. There were dozens of runners warming up running around the track, so I approached the first person I saw who was standing still and asked him who I should talk to about joining the club. To his credit, and to the credit of nearly every runner I've met, he was kind, welcoming, and pointed me to the coach. I introduced myself and was invited to join in with the evening's session and see how I felt.

I have no idea what the session was, but I do remember it being a beautiful sunny evening. To start with we all jogged easily around the track to warm up followed by the coach leading the big group in some dynamic movements. I had never heard of dynamics. High knees, heel flicks, straight leg kicks, skipping, bounding, all kinds of new exercises. There were plenty of people doing these prior to the races I had been at, but I always thought, "Is this what runners actually do before they run?" Well, it turns out it is. After we completed the session, there were a couple of easy laps to cool down and then stretching. There was also quite a bit of chatting and laughing too. I didn't get talking to too many others, but I could tell there was friendship among these clubmates. Running is a bond that each of these people had in common. I missed the team sports I used to play in the States and liked the look of this. Maybe this was what my life had been missing for the last twelve years.

The club met every Monday evening and after that first session, I just couldn't wait to get back to the next one. This second session was even more memorable. It was a remarkably warm summer evening in Fermanagh, bordering on hot, sunglasses weather. We met at the track and did our warm up as a jog to a local rugby pitch where we were instructed to remove our shoes. We did two minutes on, one minute off, barefoot on the grass. Barefoot running has since become one of my staple workouts as I enjoy it so much. The added bonus is that it promotes much better running form. I don't think I ever ran with so much enthusiasm or put in so much effort during this workout. I was learning what proper training was all about and I was loving it. On top of the great session, a couple of runners got chatting with me during the warm up. They made me feel part of the group and showed me what the club was all about. To this day, these two are still very good friends.

At this point in my life, I worked out of the house and our business was still doing quite well. I had engineers covering most of the calls so I only had to hit the road on the odd day when there was too much work for the team to handle. At 5:45 every Monday evening, I would throw on my running gear, rain or shine, and drive the 15 miles into town. This would remain my Monday ritual for several years. The sessions were hard and challenging, the runners were friendly and fun, and I was personally finding a place in this community.

During these first few months my running improved dramatically. We did speed sessions and trained consistently. It took dedication and desire to improve and I was so enthusiastic that it was like I had never run before joining up. At this point I was forty-five years old and newly indoctrinated in the sport. I finally called myself a runner instead of just someone who runs. It did take a while before I would meet up with other clubmates for runs outside of the Monday sessions, but that was soon to follow. I got talking with other runners and got tips for training, racing and about all the running gear. It was an entirely new world, and one that I relished.

Up until this point, I would arrive at a race, sign up, get my number and show up on the start line in time to go. Who knew warming up would make such a difference. I had been asking myself, "Why is the first mile always so hard?" Well now it was obvious. I hadn't been warming up properly, or at all for that matter. When I did a proper warm up before the start, that first mile was no longer my first mile. Another thing that joining the club brought me was an understanding of pace. Running at a consistent pace, or at least a consistent effort, and having an idea what pace I should be running, depending on the distance, is so important. These points were really interesting and started to click in my head. We also worked on running technique, cadence, and breathing. There were many different styles of training and many different perspectives on trainers and kit. We were all like-minded and had a genuine interest in all things running related.

Until joining the club, I had no idea that training should consist of varying types of runs either. Learning the lingo took some time, but there was always someone there to explain the different sessions and what exactly we were trying to get out of each one. Intervals, tempos, progressions, fartleks, hill reps, recovery runs, long slow runs, the options were many. All of these runs serve a different purpose and they were introduced into training over weekly and monthly training plans. Running on different surfaces also made a difference. There was the track, the road, trails, grass, and cross-country options. By changing it up, there was a reduced injury risk as well as the added bonus of keeping things interesting. The Sunday long runs always drew a big group out, and I always got into conversations with everyone before reaching the end.

It's a wonderful thing, progress, and each of these training sessions was another step in the right direction. They built momentum and once on the upward trajectory, improvement became a compulsion; a healthy addiction. It seemed like every race I was running would prove to be another personal best. Every year I would set target goals and every year I was hitting them. It had such a positive psychological effect. I was feeling about as good as I've ever felt and I think you will find a large proportion of runners will say the same thing. It is a sport with massive mental health benefits on top of the physical conditioning.

Other clubmates were interested in seeing everyone else succeed. Some members were pacing others to new PB's. It's hard to underestimate the benefits of being part of a running club. It is literally for everyone, because no matter where you are with your running, the club atmosphere is beneficial.

Good quality shoes made distance running more manageable. This is probably the most expensive piece of kit in the sport and with so many running friends now it was easy to get trusted reviews of the new gear. This was when new trainers would cost about £100, but when the new fleet of carbon plated trainers with the latest cushioned foam technology were first coming out, there was no end to the opinions. As they became the new normal, finding the right one wasn't easy. Considering the price of trainers, it's important to get trusted opinions before splashing out £250 on a new pair.

In addition to proper training sessions, better technique and all the rest, I was introduced to more beneficial post run cool down and stretching exercises. These are important for the recovery aspect. Those days of running 10 miles and not being able to walk for hours afterward are long behind me now. There would be endless other habits I picked up from the club that never would have crossed my mind. Foam rollers became my friend and friends recommended that I find a good sports massage therapist, especially if marathons were going to be part of the programme. Hydration, nutrition, in-race fuelling was all new to me from a racing standpoint. It was vitally important, for longer races anyway, to experiment with gels and other fuel. Finding the right nutrition that sat well in my stomach took a lot of practice. I had to figure out not only what to take, but when to consume it. Everyone has their own opinion and that is down to the fact that every human body is different. I know what and when to take onboard for me, but I'd be reluctant to recommend it to anyone else because we don't all respond the same way to these things. What sits well in my stomach may initiate a gastric explosion in someone else's. For me, though, before a run, I liked to keep it simple, white carbs before a run and a mix of lean protein, complex carbs and healthy fats afterwards. During a long run, I was using High-5 gels, and I'd take them every 45 minutes, alternating between ones with caffeine and ones without.

For the first time since moving to Ireland, I felt like I was part of something. I knew people and had something to talk about with them. And, sweet cheeses, could we talk about running. I felt great about myself and proud of the improvements I was making. Much like the bathroom scale where I could see the weight coming down, I could now see my race times coming down. Both of these things were equally gratifying.

My social circle was expanding and it didn't just stop with my club, it extended to the greater running community. I got to know runners from all over Ireland. I got to visit out of the way parts of the country. It opened up new friendships that extended beyond running as well.

So far, I had tackled my physical fitness problem. I managed to get back to financial security. I had a new and improved social life. Yet, despite all these things I still had my issues. Although running had changed my life for the better, I wouldn't have said I was a terribly happy man. I still didn't have the patience to deal with situations when even the slightest thing went wrong both personally and professionally. I envied those around me who had a more positive outlook and appeared happier in themselves. I simply didn't like myself a whole lot and I blamed my circumstances. Worst of all, I didn't know how to turn that around.

THE PATH TO PROGRESS

Anyone who takes up this sport will likely improve quickly as long as they train consistently. However, I don't believe I would have ever come as far as I did if it wasn't for the amazing people I met through the club. I never would have set the goals I did, or had the confidence to chase them. The people, the positive experiences, the improved fitness, as well as the ongoing healthy lifestyle is down to this club as well as the greater running world.

Good habits developed and early results both encouraged me and helped nurture a growing love for the sport. Building confidence and a positive mindset is as important in running as is talent and hard work. A runner with self-belief is more likely to be a successful runner, mostly because that is the ultimate reward even beyond running a personal best. These days a PB for me now may mean taking a few seconds off of a 5k, and those few seconds are probably more hard earned than a few minutes were in the first couple of years. The races below are some examples of the effects of that hard work and consistent training and even more so, the personal growth experienced from racing.

HOMETOWN RACE

Nobody really knows how fast they can run until they get comfortable being extremely uncomfortable. I know it sounds obvious, but our bodies won't do more than they can do, but most likely, can do a lot more than we imagine possible. This first year of structured training was amazing and progress was rapid. After only a few weeks I was running as a member of my new club at the local Enniskillen 10k, an annual event put on by the town council, and my first race wearing a club vest. This race covers the town of Enniskillen fairly well, but it hits a couple of hills that will test anyone. Included in this course is a narrow path that zig-zags its way up a steep incline with several switch-backs on what's called the Ardhowen hill. It is at the start of the last mile of the race when your legs are heavy already and the climb seems endless. Once at the top of the path, the climb continues for another fifty metres before offering some slight relief with a short downhill. After another half mile, there is a sharp downhill section before it flattens out and the last 100 metres involve another set of switchbacks on the bridge over the river Erne. All the twists and turns slow everyone down just when you want to put on the big sprint finish. It's not a fast course, but I wouldn't have known a good course from a bad one.

The race takes place at 2 o'clock in the afternoon on what is inevitably the hottest day of the year in Fermanagh. There tends to be some spectators along the road in the last mile who show some compassion for the runners and have their garden hoses spraying those who need a little relief from the heat. I wasn't one of those in need of the shower, but I was running hard. I gave it all I had over the bridge and crossed the line to a greeting from some other Enniskillen Club members who finished well ahead but stuck around to support everyone else coming over the line.

After only a few weeks of good training and taking all the advice I could get from my new clubmates, I completed the course in 47:06. Getting under the 50-minute mark, especially on such a hard course, was an incredible feeling. I can honestly say I didn't see that coming and had no idea I had it in me. I was getting comfortable being uncomfortable. That was over 11 minutes better than my first 10k and a dramatic personal best. It was a big achievement for me and pointed me in the right direction for future 10ks.

THE FIRST OF MANY

The end of October every year brings about two events in my life, my birthday and the Dublin City Marathon. My first Dublin Marathon took place in 2013. This would be my fourth marathon of the year. I felt like my training had been going well and Dublin is always a big event for our running club. It was such a good feeling to go and represent the club as part of a group of seven who took part in the event. It would prove to be a great experience and of all the races I'd taken part in thus far, this was beyond anything I'd seen. The support, the organisation, and the sheer size of the event was awe inspiring.

It is special to a lot of Irish runners and not just because it is the national championship race that often determines Olympic qualification. It simply brings out the best of the city. The number collection at the expo was new to me and I really enjoyed the buzz of the crowd browsing all the stands offering the latest in running kit and advertising upcoming races. It's a good start when you are enjoying the race a full day before the starting gun goes off.

The weather was clear and dry on Marathon Monday, the October Bank Holiday in Ireland. The day began with a bag drop, where thousands of people meandered into Merrion Square to leave their race bag at its appropriate pen. These were broken down by bib number and seemed like a highly organised affair. The bag drop is literally around the corner from the finish line, making its retrieval upon race completion simple, which is much appreciated.

Once I left my bag, I followed the correct route to the corral from which my wave was slated to start. Volunteers working the race were everywhere, ensuring we did this as smoothly as possible. There were some side streets some runners were using to take some strides or just to jog around to keep warm. There were additional portaloos available and the queues stretched dozens deep at each one.

As the clock ticked down and got closer to the firing of the starting gun, the morning strip show began. Runners peeled off old track bottoms and well-worn sweatshirts and threw them with abandon to either side of the road. Everyone aimed for the footpath, but the odd garment blindsided some poor soul across the face. That year, with three waves and over 12,000 runners, the corrals were packed. Each wave was scheduled to start fifteen minutes apart. Everyone tried to get as close to the front as possible, which meant I was literally shoulder to shoulder with thousands of others. The chat was generally light hearted with everyone in good cheer and full of nervous energy. The benefit of the packed start line was that the collective body heat generated some warmth. Although the Dublin weather in October is generally dry and sunny, the mornings can be bitterly cold and this was what was on offer that morning.

Then the time finally came, the clock reset to 0:00:00 and the gun went off. The mass collection of humanity began to slowly shuffle their way towards the timing mats under the start gantry. Inevitably, there was a start, stop, start routine as everyone was anxious to get out of the pack and get their own space, but there just wasn't enough road space to allow for it. But soon within the first few hundred metres, the field began to spread out and I found a bit of room to begin the long trek to the finish line.

The route took us through the city centre and along St. Stephen's Green and followed the river Liffey before it crossed that and headed for the beautiful Phoenix Park. This part of the course was lovely, however, there were a couple pinch points, as thousands of runners entered through the gates and upon leaving, had to find a way through the exit gates on the other side. It wasn't all that bad, but it did disrupt my momentum a little. Inside the park was a pretty, green landscape with open fields, big trees and thousands of spectators offering their support. It is a common spot for family members and friends to cheer on their runners. Phoenix Park also offered the odd wee hill to contend with.

The route then took us out to Castleknock where it turned again and at mile nine took us back into Phoenix Park for a little over a mile. Upon leaving there, it was back over the Liffey and into some of the leafier parts of the city. The autumn colours on the trees and the blue sky above made this a particularly pretty section of the race as I passed by Kilmainham Gaol. At no point was the course a lonely affair and not just because of all the runners.

I was getting a good tour of the city and the support on the streets was next level. Each and every turn, every tree lined road and city street, was packed with spectators cheering everyone on. There were musicians strategically placed around the city that gave us all a big lift as we passed them. There was also one well-meaning, but remarkably untalented, drummer who caused a little distress to some, with a runner or two mumbling what they'd like to do with his drums. But for the most part, the atmosphere around the city was amazing. The water stops and gels on the course are all located at just the right points.

The course was fair with its ups and downs, as it wound its way through the city towards Merrion Park. At the halfway point, I crossed the Grand Canal before turning again, back towards the city centre. I passed Bushy Park at mile 18, Rathgar at mile 19, and Milltown at mile 20. It was here that I just wanted to stop and sit down as I had hit the wall for the first time in a race. My pace had slowed considerably, but I kept up something resembling forward momentum. The encouragement of the crowd, and of other runners as well, made stopping an impossibility and I struggled on. At the end of mile 22 was the biggest and most energy sapping hill on the course, but why would it be anywhere else? This part of the circuit was loaded with supporters coaxing everyone up this hill, offering loads of inspiration. Despite my desperate state, I arrived at the top and turned left, where I was blessed with a nice stretch of relief down the hill. Just what I needed.

Mile 24 is run on the Stillorgan Road, which is a main thoroughfare, but I soon turned right on Nutley Road, then the Merrion Road. Before too long, there was a sign marking 800 metres to go and I don't think I've ever been so happy to see a sign. However, 800 metres seems like a lifetime when it's the last half mile of a marathon. As I approached the final 400 metres, I was surrounded by massive crowds on the footpaths, and that incredible noise carried me the rest of the way to the finishing funnel, where I collected my medal, my t-shirt and a whole boatload of congratulations from volunteers, spectators, and fellow runners.

I had managed to shuffle the final six miles and I did finally manage to reach the finish line with a time of 3:49:57. There is such a fine line between pushing too hard and not pushing hard enough. On this day, I greatly miscalculated my pace and paid the price. The result was still a little more than a half hour improvement from my first marathon in less than a year, and an eight-minute personal best. I think anyone would be happy with that and I certainly was. This one would, however, act as a valuable lesson in marathon running. Train to run for an achievable time and trust your training, but don't deviate too far from the plan. I went out too hard, too fast and suffered. It was a successful day, but could have been much better.

The bag drop area was, by this time of the day, in the shadows, as the tall buildings alongside blocked out the sun and created a cold environment. One of the funniest things to behold is watching someone who has just finished a marathon attempt to insert their legs into a pair of track bottoms. If you throw in cold hands, it doubles the amusement. I was almost helpless upon finishing, and it required a monumental effort to put my warm clothes on while sitting on the cold stone steps opposite the bag drop while a chilly wind blew, further complicating matters. Eventually, I got changed and started the long walk to the pub to meet up with friends. Dublin is a globally recognised city of culture, meaning there is a lot to see and do. It is a city famous for fun nights out, great music, singing and dancing. The post-race celebrations were great fun. Sharing my experience with fellow runners and enjoying the post marathon pain has turned into an annual past-time.

CHAPTER 7
CHASING DREAMS

IN SPRING OF 2014, there were some whispers in the club about a group considering the Boston Marathon the following year. A few of us were keenly interested. Along with Roisin and I there were six more ERC members. I had all the right connections to bring a group over, give them some hometown hospitality and show them what the city had to offer. However, at the age of 45, I would need to qualify with a time of 3:25 or better. As Boston takes fastest qualifiers first, this would mean I would need to be well under that mark in all likelihood. With my personal best sitting at 3:49, I had my work cut out for me. I wasn't too confident that I could accomplish this time, but everyone in this group was sure it could be done, given the right training. That was all the encouragement I needed, and I set the goal to run a BQ (Boston Qualifier) before the cut-off date.

We had until the end of August 2014 to run a BQ if we were to have the opportunity to run in 2015. There were a few from this group of eight who had already run BQ's, but five of us still needed it. We set a target for June 1st, at the Walled City Marathon in Derry.

I was reading plenty of books on marathon running, trying to learn as much as possible. Someone recommended a training plan online that they had once used, so that was my starting point. The plan was a 16-week training programme aimed at someone training for a sub 3:30 time. It consisted of a wide range of sessions and included upwards of five to six days of running per week. It maxed out at 60 miles in a single week. I eagerly got started, gradually building up the Sunday long run, peaking at a 22 miler four weeks out. I found these long, slow runs were by far the most enjoyable, much more so than the intervals on the track.

Winter is a tough time of year for training with the shortened daylight hours and cold, wet and miserable weather. There were some lonesome nights on the track in the pouring rain where there must have been people in their warm, dry cars driving by thinking, "What kind of moron would be out running in circles on a night like this?" The answer was I was that kind of moron. The work needed to get done and the plan had to be followed.

Late into week 3, I raced a local 10 miler and finished in a time of 1:13:42. When looking that up in *The Competitive Runner's Handbook*[1] in their "Goal Setting and Race Time Prediction" table, this would equate to a 3:27:14 marathon finish. In just week three with 13 weeks to go, that was, without question, a positive sign.

However, when week five rolled around, I pulled up on Tuesday with a pain in the front of my leg, from the top of my foot to midway up the shin. Over the next few days, the pain got worse. It started to swell and it was a struggle to lift my toes with my heel on the floor. After a visit to the physio, it was diagnosed as a strained tibialis anterior. That was both good and bad news. It wasn't so serious that I'd be out for an extended period, but I would miss some training. I lost a total of five weeks of running and it set the plan back greatly. During those five weeks, I missed three runs of twenty or more miles. This was truly the heart of the programme. I would have to make adjustments to stay on course, or at least make it to the start line in some kind of shape.

After five weeks off, in week eleven I managed 28 miles of the 60 that was on the schedule. Not great, but at least I was back running pain free once again. In the sixteen weeks, I ran 463 miles of the 746 pencilled in. Injuries happen, and it is disappointing when they do, but it is part of all sports. It left me with little confidence that such a significant improvement from my previous time was now going to be possible. I hadn't found my positive internal voice yet, and wasn't aware that I needed to conquer self-doubt in order to run my best. What I did have was good advice and the grit and determination of somebody with a purpose. I wanted to run the qualifier for all my friends planning on a trip to Boston, but I also wanted to prove to myself that I was good enough. The plan came to an end and we lined up for our target race.

WELCOME TO THE WALLED CITY

The day had come. June 1st rolled around a bit too quickly for my liking, considering my lost training weeks, but I had managed to complete the last six weeks of the programme. I needed to improve my marathon time by twenty-five minutes if the day was to be considered a success. We drove up to Derry with some friends in the morning and made our way to the bus, which took us to the hotel where the race headquarters and start line was located.

My circumstances had left me with very low expectations, but I still needed to push myself to the limit. At the very least I felt I should be able to run a PB, even if it wasn't a qualifier. My nervousness was evident as I left my gels in the car and was on the bus to the start line before I realised it. Luckily, a friend had brought extras and she gave me a few of hers, as well as an armband to carry them in. That was one disaster averted.

The five of us from Enniskillen hoping to run a BQ lined up side by side. As we stood on the start line, Martin McGuinness officiated the ceremonial start. Whatever anyone thought of him and his politics, he proved to be a very charismatic man and he had most of us laughing, which relieved some of the pre-race tension. It wasn't a huge field at the start line as race entries were capped at 1,500.

For the first few miles, we ran in a small group and kept together. After about three miles, the group started to break up into our respective paces. This was a tough enough course with a few difficult climbs in it. It left the city for a few miles and climbed up some long drawn-out hills. The one at mile 10 is probably the longest pull, and it taxed my legs, which made me question my condition. I made my way back into the city, finding a nice downhill along the way, which made amends for the difficulty going out. The course flattened out for a while along the old railway line which, along with the downhill section, allowed me to make up for some lost time. While out on the country roads, the support was rather quiet, but as you approach the signature part of the course that is turned on its head.

I say the hills are generally tough, but none nastier than the one coming at the end of mile 25, Fahan Street, the course's defining moment. I say it is nasty, but it is also the one part of the race that makes it stand out from all other races. As I ascended this section of the course, I found myself literally running the gauntlet of supporters. There was a huge crowd on either side of the street, which gave runners a path maybe five feet across to get up. The cheering was loud, there was live music, drums banging, and a cacophony of noise. I knew if this didn't propel me up the hill, nothing would. I loved every gruelling step. All the spectators were screaming and telling me how great I was doing. This particular part of the route is what would bring me back to this race again.

After I reached the top of Fahan Street, it was a good long stretch of runnable downhill and flattened out as I made the final left turn to the finish line in Guildhall Square. Once again, I finished a marathon with a PB, beating Dublin by thirteen minutes. Unfortunately, it was not a Boston Qualifier at 3:36:08. I still had eleven gruelling minutes to shave off. Considering the missed training, I was still very pleased with this result. However, if I was to make Boston in 2015, I had better do some improving, and quickly. On the more positive side, each of the others looking for a BQ got their time and did so with plenty of room to spare. Out of the eight Enniskillen runners looking to run Boston, I was the only one still chasing my time and there was only three months left in order to get it.

BEWARE OF THE VIKINGS

The search for the next eligible BQ race began, and it proved to be down in Waterford, some 225 miles south of Fermanagh, taking place on June 28th. I had four weeks to make myself ready, but having just run one, the first couple of weeks were mostly recovery.

Waterford is a very nice city and the Waterford Viking Marathon is hard to fault. The weather was shaping up to be a hot, sunny day on the south coast. Roisin and our friend Siobhan decided to run this as well, so we were going back on the road for another wee adventure.

This was a relatively small event with only 375 runners taking part. For a city marathon, the support on the street was nothing like Dublin, or even Derry for that matter, but running out to Tramore Beach and back was beautiful, and particularly nice in the bright sunshine. The temperature got up to 26 degrees, so this was by far the warmest one yet and to be honest, that sun felt great on my shoulders. There was plenty of water on the course and I made sure to take some at every station. As I strode out the Tramore Road towards the beach, and where the race turned back to the city, there were some spots where most of us managed to find some shade along the tree lined road. Otherwise, the closer to the beach we got, the more exposed to the sun we were.

Coming back towards the Waterford Institute of Technology (WIT), where the race finished, I was feeling the fatigue. The hamstrings had been complaining for a couple of miles, but now the calves were starting to knot up, letting me know they were still there. The sweat was leaving caked salt on my everything. With two miles to go, another runner made a comment to me about my club and joked that a certain member wouldn't be impressed if I slowed down this close to the finish. It turned out he was from County Clare but we had a mutual friend running for ERC. It's a small world, well Ireland is a small country anyway.

The race finished on the track at the Waterford Institute of Technology. I crossed the line and slowed down to a walk and then something unexpected happened. I had no idea what it was, but I fell to my knees and couldn't get up. Roisin says she remembers seeing me cross the line and then she blinked and I was gone. My head was spinning and my heart rate had plummeted, or so I was told later on. There was a medic at the finish line and he administered first aid right there at the track before helping me into a wheelchair. I was brought to the medical tent where I spent the next two hours tended by a doctor, nurses and physios, not to mention the slightly concerned and slightly amused Roisin and Siobhan. I was in a pretty bad way for a while. The most amusing part of this whole ordeal was that Shane, the guy who chatted to me on the course about finishing strong, was wheeled into the medical tent only a few minutes after me. There are official race photos of each of us in our wheelchairs looking like pensioners wrapped in foil blankets on one of the hottest days of the year.

I had a drip put in and the doctor was concerned about my liver function. I was grey in colour and each of my legs were spasming in turn. There was talk of sending me to the hospital, but eventually I started to come around and they let me recover where I was. The cramps subsided and I was feeling much better. The only thing stopping us from getting on our way was that we just couldn't find anyone to take the drip line out. Fortunately, Siobhan is a trained medical professional and they released me in her care with the PICC line still in. She thought it was advisable to leave it in until we got to the car just in case something happened between leaving the tent and arriving at the car. Indeed, nothing happened and I was able to walk, gingerly as you would after running hard for all those miles, to the parking lot where I sat down and Siobhan removed it. Upon removing it, she commented on my clotting ability as there was hardly any bleeding when it was removed. Not two seconds later I started gushing blood out of the wee hole like a stuck pig. She put pressure on it immediately and it stopped within minutes, but that was something we still laugh about today.

Lots of people experience hardships during and after a marathon and so when someone struggles it doesn't really raise too many alarm bells. Whether it is dehydration, muscle cramps, heat exhaustion or whatever, 26.2 miles is a long way to go and your body needs to be ready for it. In hindsight, this one makes more sense now knowing what was going to happen in less than 24 months, but there was no way of knowing there and then what was to come. Overall, this was an awfully tough way to finish a race, but I left everything on the course. My time was another PB, of almost seven minutes, and it was my first time under 3:30, but still not quite what I needed for Boston, finishing in 3:29:35. I was getting closer, but there were only two months left. Tick-tock.

A TRUE TEAM EFFORT

There isn't much chance for copious amounts of training between marathons when running them so close to each other. Considering the issues I experienced after Waterford, I had some concerns about the next one, but I needed a BQ and there wasn't a lot of time left. Taking into account some recovery time, there were still a few weeks in which to convert some good sessions, so I set to work. In order to gauge how my training was coming along, I took part in a 10k in Donegal at the beginning of August. I ran a PB with a time of 42:36. It caught me off guard as

I wasn't expecting a two-minute improvement from my last 10k. As a matter of fact, the race predictor chart worked out that this 10k time should equate to a 3:20:00 marathon time. The result got my confidence up to an all-time high and brought me into my next marathon in a good place mentally. This was going to be the last opportunity I would have to run a BQ within the qualifying window. I headed for Longford Town on August 24th for the annual Pat the Baker Longford Marathon.

This was known as a fairly flat course, but not a particularly scenic or well supported run. I had nearly two months to both recover from Waterford and to prepare for this one. I only needed another five and a half minutes of improvement and I was determined to do it. I was getting desperate. In an uncharacteristic move for me, I reached out to some of my new running friends. I asked three clubmates if they would pace me around the course in turns to keep me going and see if they could get me over the line in time. They were happy to help and I was pleased to get it.

I set off with the first runner, Rory, taking the first five miles. Rory is one of those guys who is passionate and a terrific motivator. He's also been acknowledged as a fantastic pacer in the years I've known him. I couldn't have asked for a better start. Roisin drove around the course with the team and when it was time to swap pacers, the next one would get out and the previous runner would get in the car. Talk about a team effort.

The second runner, Brian, another good friend and a fellow Boston Marathon hopeful, ran with me for the next 17 miles. He, like Rory, was amazing and kept my head strong through mile twenty-one. That was a big commitment for a pacer and so far, so good. We got through the majority of the course, which is rural and quiet on roads that are open to traffic. There was the occasional tractor that had to be negotiated, as it made its way along the narrow back roads. It was living up to its reputation as a flat course though, and that was certainly appreciated. What a benefit to have someone by my side, making sure I had water and gels when I needed them.

Between the first two pacers I was bang on target but I was hitting the most difficult part of the race. When the third pacer, Eamonn, took his turn for the final four-plus miles, I was really feeling the pain. It was getting harder and harder to take each stride but Eamonn was the right man for the job in this last push to the end. He was keeping a couple of strides ahead, taking the wind for me and was a huge help offering the advice and encouragement I needed as we approached the final stretch. He was not going to let me fail and as we turned left onto the final corner into Longford town centre, there was a larger crowd at the finish line and they were making an enormous racket. The one voice I could hear above all the others was Rory, shouting to the rest of the team, "Here they come!" Literally, over the din of the crowd I could hear that. I couldn't see him, but there was no mistaking who was shouting. Eamonn peeled off the course as I entered the finish line funnel and crossed the line in a time of 3:24:33.

I've run better times since that day, but this one will stand out in my mind as one of the most memorable days in my running life. I will forever be thankful for all of these great people. There are some running events which are a team effort, relays and cross country for example, but this wasn't normally what you would call a team event. However, the entire team, from Roisin to the pacers, all played their part to make this happen. It would never have been possible without the contribution of everyone there. This was my third PB in the space of three months, this one being just over five minutes better than Waterford at the end of June. That marked a total of 25 minutes off my marathon time from just 10 months earlier. To say I was proud would have been the understatement of the year.

The big question that would be answered in the near future: was this enough? I was only 27 seconds under the qualifying time. Over the past number of years, the actual selection times had come down. Since the Boston Marathon bombing in 2013, the number of entries for the race had climbed and it was getting harder and harder to get into. Running a BQ wasn't a guarantee of an entry, so the waiting game began.

I GOT IT, NOW WHAT?

I successfully submitted my entry for the 2015 Boston Marathon, as did the other seven local hopefuls. My entry was the only one in question as the rest of the group were well under their qualifying times. When the entry results came back from the Boston Athletic Association, I was the only one out of the eight of us who didn't make it. The cut-off time for male 45's was 3:23:57. I missed it by 35 seconds. It was heartbreaking. Could I have found 35 seconds on the course in Longford? Possibly, but I can't imagine where. I had given it all I had and at the finish line I was spent. I'll admit that I was feeling a bit sorry for myself after this huge disappointment. I would have to settle for playing host to good friends and take pride in showcasing the city where I grew up.

I explored all the avenues and tried what I could to secure a place. I reached out and applied to join three different charities, but those places for Boston were extremely hard to come by that year and I was turned down on all three applications. No doubt this was due to the increased demand as runners continued to show solidarity with the city. I told myself that it would be enjoyable enough to support my wife and the others and be there when they crossed the finish line at the pinnacle of all marathons. Boston is the oldest consecutively run marathon race in the world, first run in 1897 and still a firm favourite for many in the running world. As my friends trained for Boston, I too kept training as well in order to prepare for a spring marathon of my own. If I didn't qualify to race Boston in 2015, I was going to make sure to get there in April 2016, but as a lonesome cowboy.

CHAPTER 8
COACHING

HAVING GAINED SO MUCH from the sport, I felt I had something to give back. In the summer of 2014, the club had the opportunity to send some members to do a one-day Leaders in Running Fitness course with Athletics NI, and I volunteered to take part. This course showed the basics of how to lead a session that had been prepared by a coach. It is an important position in a club, as it covers insurance requirements and allows some structure to training sessions, particularly when a coach isn't present or when the larger group is broken up into smaller groups for separate sessions.

I mentioned earlier that I am your classic introvert, but running has given me the confidence to speak up and to lead groups of runners, coach individuals, as well as plan and deliver sessions. This was a small first step in becoming a Coach in Running Fitness, a qualification I obtained in 2015. Since doing all the work and completing the training to become a coach, I've worked with three different clubs, coaching adults and children and hopefully inspiring hundreds of runners during that time.

I've always felt that my job as a coach was to spark that bit of self-belief in someone who, until then, lacked it. Some of the most rewarding experiences in coaching for me come from bringing along new runners in *couch to 5k* programmes. The people who generally attend these programmes tend to really want to start, but find it hard to do on their own. It is so much easier to start and keep it going as part of a group, particularly when led by someone who has done it themselves.

There comes a specific moment in a 5k programme when you can see in the eyes of the participants when they first realise that they will be able to run 5k. It's about half way through, and I tell them that they have just run 10 minutes without stopping, and in this particular session, they do that twice. Once that spark is lit, doubt lifts and new runners are born. Every time I see this it brings me back to the day I first completed the entire lap at Jenkin Lakes and the incredible satisfaction it brought me as a new runner. There is no feeling like it, nor is there anything more satisfying for a coach. For many, like myself, this is the life changing experience they need and it can lead to dramatic changes in lifestyle as well as improved health and wellbeing.

Another rewarding aspect of coaching that has brought me so much satisfaction is when I have an athlete who has struggled to reach a specific goal. I take great pleasure in guiding them on their path to achieving something they thought might be beyond them. Whether that is to run under a 30-minute 5k, a 45-minute 10k, or sub three hours in the marathon, it doesn't matter. The achievement is relative to the person and what they believed unattainable. It goes beyond putting the plans together. It sometimes involves adjusting the plan, and always includes building confidence and trust.

I've been fortunate to coach young athletes and watch them

grow into amazing young adults, excelling in life and the sport. The most important thing a coach can do for a young athlete is push them to train hard, but not to the point that they don't enjoy it. There is a fine balance to strike. This is key for all athletes, but for juniors, learning to race can be the most rewarding activity they can take part in. When coached carefully, the sport helps to develop mental strength, self-confidence, and self-esteem; all of which helps to make healthy, well-rounded individuals.

CHAPTER 9
LOSING A GOOD FRIEND

WHILE GROWING up in our Massachusetts town of Stoughton, I was part of a tight group of friends who did everything together. One of the guys in this group was Tim Bulger. "The Bulge," as he was affectionately known, was a year ahead of me in school, but we grew up in the same neighbourhood, played sports together, worked together, and hung out on an almost daily basis.

In 2015, Tim had routine heart surgery to repair AFib. He went into St. Elizabeth's Medical Center in Boston, for a procedure called a catheter ablation. This is where the surgeon goes through the femoral artery in the groin with multiple catheters to create scars in the heart tissue with heat where arrhythmia is occurring. Tim had the surgery about two weeks prior to the 2015 Boston Marathon, and word spread around our group of Stoughton friends that all seemed to go well and he was recovering. He had returned home and everything seemed OK. He didn't feel great, was tired and felt queasy, but I suppose anyone would feel like that after such a procedure. After a few days he was able to go back to work on a limited basis.

Things soon turned tragic when he was rushed to hospital after collapsing at home. The emergency services were called and he was taken by ambulance to a local hospital, The Good Samaritan in Brockton, before being rushed into Boston to the Brigham and Women's Hospital where the specialists were, and was placed on life support. Things didn't improve and Tim passed away on the evening of April 22, 2015. In addition to his parents, his brother and sister, Tim left behind his wife Aimee and two young daughters, Brooke and Kate. He should have had a long life ahead of him. We all miss him, something awful.

This surgery should have been relatively straight forward. How could something like this happen to an otherwise healthy, vibrant young man? Tim worked hard, never smoked, was fit and athletic, drank very little alcohol, ate well and generally looked after himself. He was surrounded by a loving family, great friends and was well liked and respected by everyone he came into contact with. The passing of such a great person and such a close friend hit me hard. I still think of Tim often, as all his friends and family do. As a matter of fact, when we play cards, Tim is dealt into every hand, and nobody wins a hand unless they *beat The Bulge*. When I'm running and it feels hard, I remind myself of how lucky I am to be able to run, how lucky I am to wake up each morning and most importantly, how lucky I was to have had a friend like Tim to grow up with. When things are put into perspective, I have nothing to complain about. I have been very fortunate in my life and we should never take things for granted.

CHAPTER 10
THE MOTHER OF ALL MARATHONS

FRIDAY, April 17, 2015 rolled around and we travelled as a group of eight to Boston, where we all stayed at my parents' house. In the days leading up to the race, we went out for short group runs and I led everyone on a tour of Stoughton, MA, my childhood home. We had a great time and the weather was just perfect. That is, the weather was perfect the day before and the day after the marathon. The only day that really mattered, Marathon Monday, dawned with horrendous conditions. It was in the top 10 worst days in the 124-year history of the marathon. The temperature was a cold 6 degrees Celsius, 43 Fahrenheit, with driving rain and strong, icy winds. This was a tough day for competitors and spectators alike. Despite the awful weather, the people of Boston didn't disappoint. The streets were still packed with spectators and music.

My brother Kevin drove all seven participants to the drop off point, where buses took them to Athlete's Village near the start line in Hopkinton, MA. All of the runners, no matter what wave they're in, meet here and each wave is taken to their starting pen in a very organised manner. On this day there were State Police officers with high powered rifles positioned on top of the surrounding buildings at the start line. Pretty scary stuff, but they were obviously not leaving anything to chance. Security was the number one priority.

The Enniskillen runners flew around the course despite the weather, and some of them landed significant PBs. There is a family meeting area on Stuart Street where we all met up. They picked up their gear and found some space in an office building lobby where they, along with dozens of strangers, stripped down, dried off and put on fresh, warm clothes. We walked them back to our hired van, where my brother was waiting, and made our way back to his house for the post-race celebrations.

The exhausted group had sports massages booked at the house later that evening. This was a welcome treat after such a hard day. Well, maybe a sports massage can't be called a *treat*, but it certainly helped the recovery process. We all stayed there that night and enjoyed the celebrations because, after all, there were some amazing results. We moved back to my parents' house on Tuesday, when the sun blessed us with its presence once again. What a cruel joke the marathon gods played by giving the day before and the day after the race such warm and sunny conditions and sandwiching terrible weather in between.

We flew home on Wednesday, the 22nd of April. I had the opportunity to visit Tim in the hospital on the morning we travelled back to Ireland. On my visit I met his family who I hadn't seen in years and it was a sombre affair. Tim was on life support at the time, as he had been since getting taken there days before. This meant that a loud ventilator was filling his lungs with oxygen and doing his breathing for him. It was an awful hard thing to see and I truly felt for each and every one of the people who knew and loved Tim. Later that afternoon when we touched down in Dublin and I turned my phone back on, I had a message saying Timmy had passed. I had a new reason to run Boston in 2016, for Tim.

This entire episode of my life taught me so many valuable lessons. Starting with the effort it took to chase down a Boston Qualifier to the passing of a great friend. Life is not always going to go our way, and sometimes the results are just tragic. Nothing can be done about what happened in the past, however. There are only our memories to learn from and the future we aim for. The thing we have total control of is what we do today. All the preparations we make can be thrown off course in the blink of an eye. We were all going to need to find a way to cope with the loss of Tim, in our own way, and make sure his legacy lives on.

Despite running the BQ, I didn't get to run Boston with my friends. That said, the whole experience made me more determined than ever to keep improving. I knew that I would continue to make progress. I was getting to know my body better, what it responded to in training and what nutrition worked best for me. I was growing in experience and ability.

CHAPTER 11
BQ ATTEMPT 2

AFTER ARRIVING BACK in Ireland in April 2015, it took some time to get back into a routine. I was all out of sorts. It's weird when something tragic happens when you are 3,000 miles away. It's obviously not the same thing, but the feeling was something like after the 9/11 attacks in the States. I think I struggled here because there was nobody to share my grief with. There were people here who were upset, but there weren't any Americans who could understand the grief as a fellow countryman. Similarly, when I lost a loved one at home, I didn't have my friends nearby to share the loss, and therefore, it made getting over it a little bit different. Not harder but different. During these times, I felt so incredibly distant and alone.

Soon after our return, Roisin and I also sold our business. I desperately wanted to get out of the IT world and into something completely different. We started up a sports tourism company, which was more in-line with our love of running. It was slow to start, but we were confident that our past experience would be of great value and we could make this a success, much like the previous business. We put a lot of time and effort into this new venture, and we had the finances from the sale to keep us going while we tried to get this one off the ground.

Meanwhile, running makes for the perfect distraction and it is a great activity for dealing with difficult issues. Like I said previously, therapy in the form of exercise. I continued my quest to run Boston with a spring marathon. I wouldn't need to improve a great deal, but I would need to find those evasive 35 seconds at the very least. When running got tough or I was feeling tired or in pain, I had someone to think about. My pain and tiredness were nothing compared to losing a good friend. So, after a week in Boston, I put my racing head back on. I was in good shape from my spring training, and I would be fit to tackle my spring marathon and reach that all important goal.

ALONG THE TOWPATH

I chose a local marathon as my first attempt to run a BQ for the 2016 event. The window had just opened and I hoped to qualify towards the start of the window rather than wait until the last minute, like the last one. There is a qualifying marathon in Newry Co. Down. It is only a little over an hour from Fermanagh, so I had all the comforts of home. I was able to eat normally and plan my evening food much better than if I was away. My go-to carb loading meal was pizza in those days. This was the perfect meal the night before. One needs to be careful on the evening meal before race day. There is a great expression that says "the more you carb-load, the more you need to carb-unload." I am always careful to not go overboard. I also had the comfort of my own bed and made my own breakfast of porridge and toast with peanut butter. These little points make a big difference for marathon race day.

It was a cold and wet day and I arrived early along with two other clubmates also taking part, picked up our racing bibs and managed to keep warm enough waiting for the start. Just before the gun went off, the weather cleared up and left an overcast, but fairly dry and calm morning. The starting field was quite small, with only 165 lining up. It was a quiet course with very few spectators on the route other than the wonderful volunteers who marshalled and handed out water along the way. The route was decent, with a few hills and a long stretch along the canal towpath which was as flat as it gets.

Everything went to plan here and maybe I had found a good routine that would stand to me in future races. As the day warmed up the on-course, water and my gels were taken on-board according to plan. I had four gels, one every 45 minutes and water at every station along the way. I crossed the timing mat at the finish in 3:19:03. I had it, finally! Surely it would get me into Boston for 2016 and in the end it did.

A WARM WELCOME HOME

April 18, 2016 was a warm day in Boston. Not like 2015, where the city of Boston experienced horrendous conditions. This day was clear, calm, and sunny. Kevin dropped me off at the bus to take me to the Athlete's Village bright and early, which gave me time to get a coffee and relax once I was there. I laid out under the warm sun and just basked in my hard-won circumstances. This was a place many runners would love to be, and I was so fortunate to be one of the lucky ones who made it. Looking around at the crowd brought to mind my running friends and the esprit de corps of fellow athletes. And I thought about Tim, as it was almost one year ago that we lost him.

Maybe I should have put sunscreen on, but it never occurred to me. I had also forgotten plasters for my nipples so I went to the medical tent and they kindly provided me some free of charge. That's a mistake an endurance runner only makes once as the chafing can be excruciating.

Athlete's Village has coffee, tea, water, fruit, and other snacks available under a huge canopy. They also had hundreds of portaloos, which got plenty of use. The number of people were just overwhelming and although this was now three years from the tragic bombings, the pride of the city was still on display. I was a proud Bostonian for sure. When my wave was called, I joined thousands of people slowly pressing toward the correct corral, and one generous runner passed around his bottle of sunscreen, which as an Irishman, I greatly appreciated.

Today was a run for Tim. I remember that while going around the course, memories would flood back to when we were kids. The hours spent playing street hockey. The parties at his house when we were in high school. The time we spent as a big group of friends watching Boston Bruins games in his basement. The time we were on Spring Break in Daytona Beach, Florida and had enough drink for the week, so instead of continuing on to the next club, we ended up in an IHOP ordering T-bone steaks at two in the morning. The holidays down in Cape Cod where we spent so many hot summer days enjoying a BBQ and cold beers. The weekends away in New Hampshire where we had some unforgettable times at the Boxmore. Tim somehow always managed to do something that made everyone laugh and he was such an important part of our lives. So many memories came back, and I was literally in tears during a few sections of the route when something would trigger another memory. I don't know what I must have looked like.

The Boston course was a completely new experience. The first half, believe it or not, is mostly downhill, which everyone taking part should know beforehand. Knowing it is one thing but being prepared for it is something else. Going downhill for so many miles is a quad-killer. By mile 11, my quads were in bits. There is some undulation in the first half, but the sore quads caught me off-guard. However, getting closer to the halfway mark it's obvious that something special is coming up. There is noise on the horizon. It's called the *Scream Tunnel* and this is at Wellesley College, where hundreds of young women from the school are holding signs reading, "Kiss Me." It is a completely unique experience and a sensation I will never forget. No, I didn't kiss anyone, nor slow down for that matter, but the Scream Tunnel was an unforgettable, extraordinary experience that reignited my adrenaline.

The second part of the course includes more uphill terrain and is by far more of a pull on the legs. Normally, I can deal with the uphills on a course because I know there will be relief in the form of downhill on the other side. However, with the sore quads from the first half, I took no great pleasure in travelling downhill in the second. I hit the Newton Hills in miles 17 through 21, including the infamous Heartbreak Hill. This is a series of sharp hills that test even the most seasoned runners, more because of their location in the course than because of their difficulty, but they are tough enough. They drag out over five miles and the downhill recovery hurts anyway, there are very few words to describe this section of the course other than pain.

Once through this, the hardest section of the race, it does get better. The Red Sox play a morning home game every

Patriots Day, meaning that there is quite the buzz from base-ball fans as they mull about Kenmore Square, outside Fenway Park. Street vendors, and those who didn't get a ticket to the ball game, stick around to watch and cheer the runners as they pass during their last mile of the marathon. Very soon after this, I took a right hand turn onto Hereford Street and then the final left onto the famous Boylston Street. I could see the finish and the crowd was massive there, but it was a long straight-away to reach the line. This was my chance for that final push to make up a few seconds and possibly take my time under my target. As I crossed the line and stopped the watch, it was another personal best. I completed the Boston Marathon in 3:18:30.

This was a special race for me. I found the people of Boston so incredibly generous with their support. It is well known for its large Irish population, so it was heart-warming to get so many shoutouts for my Enniskillen Running Club vest. I heard many shouts of "Up Fermanagh," and "Go Enniskillen," throughout the day. I even heard my name called out from someone who I played ice hockey with thirty years earlier. Despite my white hair and mid-life wrinkles, I was still recog-nised. This personal greeting gave me a real boost. It took some willpower not to stop for a quick chat.

For the remainder of my trip, I was walking on clouds. I received congratulations from all my friends both at home and in Boston. None more than from Roisin and the kids, who knew how much effort that whole endeavour took out of me. That was a long-fought battle to gain entry and to run that race. I did it, and did it well, which was incredibly satisfying. Additionally, I got to spend time with my parents, family and friends. We also had a one-year anniversary for Tim, where all his friends and family got together to celebrate him. This was an entirely beautiful trip home and returning to Ireland wasn't going to be easy.

RACE TIMES CONTINUE TO FALL

Ever since we moved to Ireland, I experienced brief periods of low mood whenever I returned from a trip to the States. This was normal. But then in May, I experienced some issues personally. The new business just wasn't getting anywhere and I was finding this new industry far more difficult. Roisin began a job managing an office with a local start-up business. Additionally, she started taking courses for sports massage therapy. Between these two commitments, she was running less and less and her racing took a backseat. As the months came and went, and despite Roisin's job, the financial pressures were taking their toll on me and I was a bundle of nerves. This should have been a time to celebrate success, but instead, it was a time of anxiety.

Once again, running came to my rescue and offered the outlet I needed to blow off steam and think problems through to gain clarity. Although I enjoy the structured training when following a plan, there's also a freedom that comes from doing what you want, when you want. For the remainder of the spring and summer of 2016, I took part in local races of shorter distances as well as weekly Parkruns.

Parkrun is a timed, non-competitive 5k that runs every Saturday morning. Originating in the UK, they are now found in 22 countries around the world in countries like the United States, Canada, Germany, and as far away as Australia. Because my local Parkrun, in Enniskillen, is run over the same course every week, it is a great method to gauge where I am at in my training or my current fitness level. The social benefits are hard to beat too. When I'm not running it, I can often be found volunteering at it, which is what I did in the weeks following my return from Boston.

On May 7, 2016, a group of us went to Ballyshannon, in County Donegal to run a 5k. I knew, going in, that physically I felt good coming off a successful run in Boston the month prior. The course was undulating for the first 2.5k, and then levelled off with a nice downhill finish along the water. When I got over the line and stopped the watch, it showed 18:11. By far my best time in a 5k with a huge PB by over a minute. After that, 5K's became my second favourite distance.

Then in August, once again in County Donegal, this time in Lifford, I ran my first sub 40-minute 10k finishing in 39:35. Maybe I should have moved to Donegal?

I had managed to reach some of the target times many runners aim for. It was a very successful year of running for me. My next goal was to qualify for the London Marathon. For me that would mean running under 3:15. At the time, if you ran a good-for-age qualifying time for London, you were guaranteed a place. So even squeaking under that time would do it. That meant I had to take another three minutes off my PB, but the way I had been improving had filled me with confidence. I was absolutely convinced I could get there.

ANOTHER VISIT TO DUBLIN

In August I started training for Dublin, and from some of the results I was posting during the summer, all the signs were good for a London qualifying time. I didn't manage to get it in Boston, but I wasn't far off and I knew I could achieve this by October. I had missed the window to qualify for the 2017 London

Marathon, but should I run a time, it would make me eligible for 2018.

When I crossed the finish line in 3:14:23, I secured my London place. I needed that bit of success more than I needed anything at that point in my life. The joy on the finish line was short lived though. Upon finishing the race, I had a bit of a brain cramp and couldn't find any of my friends and I had no idea how to get back to the hotel. I also hadn't put a phone in my drop bag, so I had no way to contact anyone. What should have taken 15 minutes took me two hours to find my way back. Part of the problem I encountered was that I couldn't cross the marathon route, so I kept being sent around strange, never before seen roads in the city. By the time I found Roisin, she had nearly all the hospitals called. Having lived through the post Waterford Marathon episode, she'd been increasingly worried. When I did manage to make it back there was a general sense of relief (and maybe a little anger). After some apologies, a shower and a change of clothes it was off to the celebrations with the rest of the finishers.

With Dublin behind me, it was time to address the rest of my problems. In November I updated my CV and started a new job hunt. I had been running my own companies since 2004 and I knew it was time to let someone else bear the burden of keeping a business above water. I would be happy to do my job and collect my wages. In December, I landed a contract position with the Cooneen Group, a company only a few miles away as an IT Manager. This had been a pretty tough year, but it was coming to a positive end. I had some room to exhale and 2017 was going to be full of optimism.

CHAPTER 12
WHAT JUST HAPPENED

I HAD big plans for the new year. I had a new job and some target races. The plan for spring 2017 was to take part in the Manchester Marathon. I'm always off to a slow start the first two weeks in January as I work off the over-indulgences of the holidays. But by the end of January, I was back to running 20 miles and ramping up the weekly miles incrementally. On Sunday the 5th of February, I ran 18 miles at a slow, steady pace and I felt strong with each one passing by easily. Little did I know how my world would change soon after that when my hopes for running my best ever marathon, in Manchester, or anywhere else, came crashing down.

Tuesday morning at 5:55 am on February 7, 2017 was cold and outside a heavy rain was falling. I climbed the stepladder to my attic where my weights and bench were located. I had created an area where I could escape in the early mornings for some strength training before heading to work. This space was directly above the bedrooms in our bungalow, meaning I tried to keep as quiet as humanly possible.

I had been running very well of late and my 5k and 10k times were all trending in the right direction, sending my confidence soaring. Additionally, I had been doing bigger miles, between 50 on the lighter weeks and 80 on the heavier ones, and I was well into a solid training block. Weight training was an important part of my plan in reaching the next level as a runner.

On this fateful morning it was to be an upper body session, working on chest and shoulders. Typically, I would do my first set of bench presses with a light weight and do 20 reps in order to warm up the muscles and then go up in weight for 10 reps, up again for 8 reps and up again for 6 reps. I started the Fitbit at 6:03 am, and away I went, the first set with just the bar went with no problems. My inexpensive gym equipment consisted of a bench that required small 3-inch pins to be inserted into the uprights when changing weights, to prevent the bar from tipping to the heavier side and dumping the weights and bar with a crash to the floor. I started to put the pins in but I dropped the left one. I bent down and lifted it, with some difficulty, and then dropped it once again. Eventually I managed to insert it using both hands and attempted to add weights to the bar. When adding the 10kg plate I dropped it, making a loud bang on the attic floor. I was sure all of this commotion must have caused great concern below. Apparently, my family sleeps much more soundly than I thought. I was expecting someone to poke their head through the access panel telling me to keep it down, but no one emerged. I bent down and lifted the plate and managed to get it on the bar, again using both hands.

I tried to make my way around to the front of the bench in order to begin the next set of bench presses but I stumbled and fell to the floor. I managed to get myself to my feet but when attempting to take another step, I immediately fell to the floor once again. I felt tired, drained. It never occurred to me that there was anything wrong. I thought I was being clumsy from over exertion. I didn't get angry or frustrated that these things were happening. The second time I hit the floor, I decided that I should just close my eyes and rest, and so I did.

It must have been a good 30 minutes later when I woke up and tried to move. Moving was hard. My body wasn't responding. I thought I should make my way back down the ladder, go back to bed and forget about this morning's workout. As it was difficult to move, I decided to try to get someone to help me down, but I still didn't mentally grasp that there was anything wrong. It's funny how the mind works, as the whole experience was dream-like.

I wasn't able to stand up, so I dragged myself along the floor about 10 feet away where my phone was on a small table and managed to reach up, grab it and ring Roisin. No answer. I tried Aidan, and once again no answer. I tried Roisin's phone again, but still no answer. I dragged myself to the access panel where the ladder was, but there was no way I was going to manage the ladder down. I didn't want to try to shout because I didn't honestly think anything was wrong with me. I also didn't want to wake Catraoine or Daniel, so I rang Roisin once again. On my third attempt she awoke and answered the phone. She saw the number was mine and asked if I was OK. I answered, "I don't know." At least that's what I thought I said. I can't say for sure what it sounded like.

At this point it was still only about 6:40 in the morning. She knew straight away something wasn't right and came up into the attic where I was laying prostrate near the access panel. She asked me to look at her and say something. My speech was slurred and only the right side of my mouth was moving. She asked me to lift my arms and I was only able to lift my right arm. To her credit, she recognised the signs of a stroke but remained calm. Yet, even though I recognised why she asked me to do those things, I still didn't think that anything serious was wrong. I thought she was crazy to even test me for a stroke. I was obviously too young, and too healthy to experience something like that.

Being a hardcore runner, my initial thought was to stop my Fitbit, which I managed to do and save the activity. Looking back on my Fitbit activity for that day showed a 43-minute workout, which actually included only one set of bench presses. I started coming around at this point and with some help was able to stand up, shakily, and Roisin summoned Aidan from his bed to assist me down the ladder. I sat on the couch in the living room for a short time, feeling fine, a little light-headed, but still absolutely convinced there was nothing wrong. I had no intention of going to the hospital but thankfully Roisin insisted and she called an ambulance. The kids thought I had just taken a fall and was taken to the hospital to get checked out. They had no idea anything more significant had happened, and went to school as normal.

County Fermanagh is a rural area to say the least. We live five miles from the nearest small town in a quiet country location that is rather difficult to direct visitors to. Roisin figured the best course of action was to meet the ambulance halfway from the hospital, which was some twenty miles away. She packed me in the car and away we went. The meeting point was in a village called Maguiresbridge where the ambulance met us and I was transferred. It was still cold and dark and wet. By this time, I felt a bit foolish to be in an ambulance as everything seemed to be working and I could talk and walk without too much trouble.

However, the ambulance workers recognised all the things Rosin described to them as stroke symptoms and they delivered me safely to the A & E department in the South West Acute Hospital (SWAH) in Enniskillen. She followed in her car.

The nurses took me in and carried out all the basic tests. I don't think there was too much panic, as I was in pretty good form by then. I had a CT scan and an ECG and they continued to monitor me for an hour or two. It's at this point I should point out that the SWAH was in the very fortunate position of having one of the best stroke units in all of the UK, headed up by Professor Kelly, an extremely caring and capable professional. After all of the initial scans, and given that I seemed to be past the worst of the symptoms, Professor Kelly recommended an Angio CT scan to get a better understanding of what happened. All the signs pointed to a TIA, a mini-stroke that clears on its own. The best way to get confirmation on this would be with this type of brain scan. It would also give a much clearer picture as to what the next steps in treatment should be.

I was taken down to the CT scanning lab in a wheelchair and parked outside the doors in the waiting area. A nurse came by to put in a new PICC line, but there was a slight issue with getting it in. Soon though, a young doctor came by and got it sorted relatively quickly and left me so he could inform the staff that I was ready for the scan at any time. As I sat in the wheelchair, all alone, and only moments after the doctor left, I had the sudden strange sensation wave over me. I lost all feeling in my left side once again. I tried to yell for help but I couldn't speak. I could only make noises. Strange and horrible sounding noises, more like loud grunting and groaning than anything. I made these noises as loud as I could, trying to get someone's attention.

That was the first time in the entire ordeal that I realised something was wrong and I will admit, I was panic-stricken. While the morning episode felt more imaginary than real, I was fully awake the second time and knew for a fact what I was experiencing. After some time, I don't know for sure how long it was, I got the attention of someone passing by. They raised the alarm and moments later, the staff lifted me out of the wheelchair and back onto a bed, and then summoned Professor Kelly and a team of doctors. They immediately identified that I was experiencing a stroke and they administered thrombolysis there and then. I was taken back to the A & E department for closer observation while the medication took effect.

When I arrived back at A & E with the medical team, Roisin was there waiting, and was informed of what was happening. There was a great weight on my chest that was causing me enormous distress. It turned out to be my left arm. Someone must have placed it there while I lay on the hospital bed, to keep it from dangling down. It felt like a ten-tonne weight bearing down on me and although I was sure it was my arm, because I could see it, I had no feeling and couldn't move it. It was like a piece of meat and it felt awful where it was. I attempted to communicate to everyone around me to have it moved off my chest, but it took ages to get anyone to understand what I wanted. Eventually, Roisin translated my grunts and groans and the offending appendage was moved and placed down by my side. I was completely helpless and scared.

Roisin left to phone family and my work to let them know what was going on. When she returned to me, she was with our friend Siobhan, who works in the hospital, had heard I was there, and came down to see how I was. This was the same Siobhan who kindly removed the line from my vein in Waterford. I don't know why, but when the two women came in to see me, I fell apart and just started crying. I still couldn't talk at this point and that probably had something to do with it. All at once, I had realised the seriousness of what I was going through, and that this wasn't going to be over any time soon. The thoughts going through my head were the scariest of all. Was I going to survive? What was going to happen to my family? Would the kids be OK without me? Will I ever be able to walk and talk again? I had just started a new job and what was going to happen there? These thoughts came a mile a minute and flooded my brain like a tsunami.

The thrombolysis worked its magic and within an hour I was able to speak again, slowly and slurred, but I could communicate. I was left a little sore and a lot confused. Over the next few hours, the results of my falling and thrashing about in my attic became a little more evident as I had a pretty good black eye and massive bruising on my arms and legs. Looking at me you'd have thought I lost in a rock fight.

Although as a child I had spent my fair share of time in the hospital emergency rooms, I had never enjoyed the hospitality of an overnight stay. Well, that's not entirely true, I was present for the birth of our four children, so technically I had been overnight, but never due to my own medical needs. I was now booked in for an extended stay in the SWAH. I was admitted and checked into a comfortable, single room to set up camp on Ward 5 for the foreseeable future. There was a heart monitor connected to me at all times which meant there was a tangle of wires attached to my chest to go along with the oxygen tubes in my nostrils and the PICC line in my left arm. All these things made movement awkward and uncomfortable. At the time my normal resting heart rate was in the low 40's and when sleeping, it dropped into the 30's. Such a low rate caused the alarms to go off regularly. It is hard enough to sleep when in the hospital but near impossible when alarms are beeping and ringing throughout the night.

For the first two days I wasn't allowed to get up and go to the toilet without letting the staff know I needed to get out of bed. It was a slow and careful walk to the bathroom which was only a couple of metres away. The number of tests and scans that were carried out over the first several days were nothing short of mind boggling. I was turned into a human pin cushion as I couldn't even begin to count the number of times I had needles put in and blood taken out. It's never been one of my favourite things, but I soon got used to it.

During these first few days, Professor Kelly was busy analysing the data from all the tests. He confirmed that it was in fact a stroke, no surprise there, but what would cause a 48 year old, with an above average fitness level, to have a stroke? My weight was a strong 165 lbs. Up to this point, I had not suffered any injuries that would have put my running back any more than a few weeks. So, what was it? Not only was our local hospital fortunate enough to have a top stroke team, the head Cardiologist is top of her field as well. Dr. Monaghan got to work putting the pieces together along with Professor Kelly.

Without question, the worst part of the entire investigation was what is called a transoesophageal echocardiogram. This is a long thin lubricated scope, like a camera, that was inserted down my throat to take an ultrasound of my heart without ribs or any other bones or tissue getting in the way. It gives the doctors a clearer picture of the heart. Even the name of it sounds awful and it certainly lived up to my expectations. I was given a local anaesthetic to numb my throat to allow for it to relax for the tube to be eased down my oesophagus. I kept gagging and choking on it and it was quite painful. I can't begin to describe the feeling. In the end they had to knock me out with something a little stronger in order to get the procedure done. After all the investigations, the doctors got what they needed and they found a 11mm hole in my heart.

Apparently, what happens when there is a hole in the heart like mine is the pressure of the heart pumping creates a rush of blood through the hole, similar to the water in a river running fast over a stone. This creates bubbles, which cause blood clots to form. In my case, these clots made their way through the hole and straight up to the brain, which caused the stroke.

The CT angiography scan was also conclusive. There was evidence of at least two blood clots that made it up into the right side of my brain, one of which broke apart and affected five additional areas.

My stroke was diagnosed very quickly and my treatment was handled with expertise. That is not the case for many people suffering a stroke. As a relatively young married man with four children, all I can do is be grateful for every day I have. There are so many what-ifs to consider. What if the NHS had closed the stroke ward in Enniskillen, like it had been threatened over the past few years? What if Roisin didn't call the ambulance and had instead listened to me on that morning when I wanted to just go to work? What if Professor Kelly hadn't been there to call for the thrombolysis as quickly as he did? The right decisions were made at each step along the way and I was fortunate.

As this was an outlier of a case, there were visits from students who would come in to talk to me, asking all sorts of questions. Nurses and doctors would come in and ask me if I was the marathon runner who had a stroke. Overall, I was treated remarkably well. The team on Ward 5 at SWAH are without exception compassionate, professional and overwhelmingly kind. I couldn't have been in better hands, and I will forever be indebted to every member of the staff there.

My physical recovery was relatively quick and I was able to walk and talk, just a little slower than before. My fitness played a part in that aspect of my recovery. There is no doubt in my mind that all the support from Roisin, my kids, extended family, friends and the entire running community that I had come to know over the past few years played a massive part in getting me back on my feet. So many people took their time to visit, and offer support either in person or by messaging me. I was grateful for all those who showed their concern and gave me their time. It really meant so much and I'll never forget it.

My stay in hospital lasted for a total of eight days and I was discharged on Valentine's Day, Tuesday the 14th of February. Unfortunately, I didn't have the time to pick up flowers or a card for Roisin. It was a happy moment when I was released and Roisin, Catraoine, and Owen, who came home from university, arrived to take me home. On the way we stopped in at Blakes of The Hollow, a local pub of some fame, for a quiet, celebratory pint of Guinness. I think we all deserved one. I was given the OK to return to running, with the instructions to keep it relatively easy for a while and to not push it too hard. This was a welcome relief to me, but it would be a long time before I was racing again.

I was prescribed two medications which are to be taken for the rest of my life. First is an antiplatelet medication called Clopidogrel. The second is a statin called Atorvastatin. My cholesterol level wasn't high to begin with, but the statin was given as a precaution and to maintain clean arteries. Some people experience issues when taking a statin with muscle soreness but, fortunately for me, I have had no issues with that. As for the Clopidogrel, the side effects are a different story. I bruise like a peach. If you look at me with side-eyes I'll be left with a contusion or two, as if a piercing stare is enough to break a blood vessel. Additionally, in the years since starting on this medication, I am always cold. This is an extremely uncomfortable way to live. I cannot get warm unless I'm sitting under a roasting sun. Otherwise, I need layer upon layer to keep comfortable. I tend to wear sweatshirts and sometimes even a woolly hat in the house. My hands seem to always be cold, even on the days when others are sweating.

During the stay in the hospital, I had so much time on my own with nothing to do. A life-threatening event like a stroke leaves you with loads of questions that loop through your head. Everything was put into perspective and I know it sounds cliché, but it changed me profoundly. As I started to feel like I was going to be OK, there were still the underlying questions as to what I would be like when I got out of the hospital. I worried that this could happen again. I wondered how I would be different from the person I used to be. Less existential worries also crept in. I was given the OK to run, but what about marathons? What about racing? I knew it wasn't overly important in the whole scheme of things, but these things were an integral part of who I had become and doubts flooded my brain. Despite the impact running had on my life up to this point, that part of me may just have to change. I was given a second chance at life. I was going to make serious changes and value the people who meant the most to me. That was first and foremost and I was determined to finally be the man I always wanted to be.

CHAPTER 13
THE AFTERMATH

FORTUNE WAS a kind mistress to me physically after the stroke. Everything physical including movement now took more effort, but I was mobile. I spent nearly every minute of the day either sitting or lying down and simple things like walking across the kitchen took it out of me. But there was no question that it was improving daily and I would continue to get better.

Without running, life would have been a much darker prospect. It was my method of keeping fit both physically and mentally. I was a little scared about going for my first run, but I knew the longer I waited, the harder it would be to conquer my fear. I got out for my first run three days after returning home with a half mile run at an 11 minute per mile pace. I was apprehensive and it felt really strange but I was thrilled to be out and doing it. My second run was another half mile two weeks later, this time at a 9:40 pace.

I wasn't able to do anything to strain myself, so weightlifting was out of the question for a while. It would be well after my heart was repaired before I could get back to it. I could live with that, as it was a small sacrifice to make in the whole scheme of things. I had four strong kids and a remarkably supportive wife. My family was understanding and helpful during this time and my recovery was in no small way expedited by the love they showed and everything they did for me. My family and friends in the USA were also a great support and it would be wrong to leave out the running groups I coached and the running friends I had made. I was coaching at two different clubs and I had a Couch to 5k programme running at the same time when this occurred. I was heavily involved in the local Parkrun, which is a great group of people who also made their well wishes known. Roisin stepped up and coached a few sessions of the beginner programme for me, which kept their progress on target while the clubs managed without me for a few weeks. I was visited at home by members of the clubs and the gifts and get well cards were much appreciated. It is hard to underestimate the importance of all of these wonderful people. The running world was there for me when I needed them the most.

Fortune, however, was not so kind to my brain after the stroke. It was hard to get a proper perspective on what the future held, and it was made even more difficult when my head was such an unmade bed. Communicating was both frustrating and exhausting. My brain felt like it was swimming around in a *word soup*. It took a great deal of effort to pluck words out of the broth and string them together into a coherent sentence. Friends and family claimed that they didn't notice much of a difference, but I am confident this was only to make me feel better. I sure noticed it. Nobody will ever understand the challenge I faced, because they never saw the internal turmoil, they just saw John. Speaking was happening in slow motion. I couldn't remember what simple everyday objects were called. This was a difficult time and the aggravation built up and would need to be released now and again. It was at these moments when an inner rage would expose itself. The smallest little thing could set me off and I would lose control of my anger at the flick of a switch. I would quickly regain my composure, but it was awful both for myself and anyone around me. I've always been impatient, but this was over the top and far more unstable. When talking to the kids about this period, later, they commented on these episodes and how uncomfortable it made them. I know it would have been a scary and unsure time for them as well. The last thing they needed was a father ready to lose his cool every time they turned around. I had promised myself I would make changes going forward, but these weren't the changes I had in mind. I wanted to take positive steps, but this was certainly a leap backwards.

Life went on around me and I witnessed it from somewhere else, almost like being in a perpetually dazed and confused state. I was also bored and lonely. After eight days in the hospital and three days home alone while everyone else was either working or at school I was getting restless. On a normal week, I'd be out getting about 40 or 50 miles running, unless training for something, and the miles would increase, but this week I had only a half mile in the bank.

Driving was out of the question for three months, and I sat home alone, way out in the countryside, in the middle of winter, no less. On Friday, February 17th, I phoned work and told them I intended on coming back to work on Monday. They were surprised and I suppose a bit curious as well, so they agreed. Fortunately, I have some very generous neighbours who I happened to work with and they were willing to take me to and from work each day.

I had only started this position in mid-December so my colleagues didn't know me too well. All they knew was that I was an active runner. The stroke took them completely by surprise as it did everyone who knew me. On Monday February 20th, after missing only two weeks of work, I returned. In hindsight, this was an extremely bad decision, one in which I was not at all ready for. I know in my heart that returning to a work environment set me back, but it was necessary to get back to work for financial reasons. As this was a contract position, I had no sick pay. Every day I missed work was another day without pay. Although that shouldn't have been a consideration, unfortunately, it was important at the time. We simply needed the money and I couldn't afford to not take home a pay cheque. For my health and well-being, I should have been off work for at least six months, maybe longer. That would have given me the opportunity for my brain to heal before frying it with work stress and responsibilities once again.

The first couple of days felt good being back at my desk, but I wasn't the same person, far from it. It took me longer to do anything than it did just two weeks earlier. Speaking, in general, wasn't easy. When I was asked a question or for an opinion, I would look the person in the eye and try very hard to first gather my thoughts and then string together the words in order to respond. It could sometimes take 10 seconds before anything could come out vocally. My self-confidence was as low as it could have been. In my mind it felt that others thought I was stupid and no longer fit for work. The harder I tried to sound like my old self, the more this seemed to confirm these feelings.

I found the general office experience tiring. Leaving work exhausted and getting home I'd collapse on the couch for a couple hours and do nothing and that was about all I had the energy for. In meetings I didn't want to engage, because speaking felt so awkward and difficult. My lovely anger issues began making appearances now and again too. I was feeling insufficient in so many ways and frustration built up until the top blew off and I either screamed or threw something. I actually did do both of those things in the office on occasion. In a flash I'd lose my head and explode at someone. People were a little more understanding afterwards, as I'm sure they knew I was struggling.

In addition to fits of rage, I was also experiencing severe mood swings. Depression would come and go. There would be days that I just didn't want to get out of bed and definitely didn't want to go to work. The moments of feeling good were always followed by those severe downturns. The good days rarely lasted longer than a few days at a time. My brain had suffered a traumatic blow and it was physically damaged. This was going to take some time to heal. I had experienced short bouts of low mood before, as I'd say most people have, but this was different. The bad days were dreadful, at times frightening for me and those around me.

My post-stroke recovery included regular visits with the occupational therapist, clinical psychologist, heart doctor and stroke doctor. I have nothing but praise for the NHS and for the way I was cared for while in the hospital. I can say the quality of the care I received during my recovery was exemplary as well. I received great help from the clinical psychologist, Dr. McKeown, who helped me with my issues of anger, rage and depression. She had such patience with me and always looked out for my best interests without pressuring me to do anything too quickly. There were some breakthrough sessions where we worked on coping techniques and mindfulness. We actually did an IQ test on one occasion and I don't think I was ever as exhausted as that, even after finishing a marathon. It completely drained me but it was incredibly interesting. I actually scored pretty well on it, with a 126, and that helped bring me forward knowing I was no more stupid than I used to be. At least I don't think so as I didn't have a previous score to compare against.

During this time, I was back to doing some running. Being able to run was a life saver. I didn't have to think about what I was doing. I was able to just lace up my trainers and go. I wasn't going to run hard or push myself too much, but putting one foot in front of the other was therapeutic. Having friends willing to join me was a big help too. A good friend, Tara Malone, was very protective and didn't want to see me running, particularly on anything resembling a pacy run, and would question whether or not I was wise to be out so soon after the stroke. Roisin wanted to ensure the medical team were fully aware of the kind of running I wanted to get back to and explained exactly how far a marathon is. But despite the concerns, I had the go ahead from both Professor Kelly and Dr. Monaghan so I was going to run. The doctors were keen for me to get back to normal life, or as close to normal as possible, and they said there was little risk of any complications from running. Particularly now that they were fairly certain of the cause and I was taking medication to prevent a recurrence.

My running was relatively slow from what I had been doing, rarely faster than a nine-minute mile. Despite the reassurances from the professionals, I was cautious, not confident in going too fast, knowing I had a rather large hole in my heart and knowing that it had most likely been the cause of the stroke. It was natural to be tentative. For the following few months, that voice no one else hears was winning the battle over my body. In

March, I took part in my first event since the stroke, the Bundoran 10k. I finished the race in 1:05:28. I wasn't chasing a time on this day. I was after a slice of normality. In that regard the day was almost a complete success.

Although I felt fine during the run, something bizarre happened when we went for food and drinks afterward. The pub we were in started filling up and got louder and louder. It was a small, enclosed environment which meant the noise was confined and bounced off the walls. It sent my head spinning. After about thirty minutes I found myself surrounded by friends while tears were streaming down my face. I was pleased to have completed the 10k, but these weren't tears of joy or of sadness. I wasn't emotional in any way, and I had no explanation for what was going on. Eventually, we left and I settled down, but this was an unwelcome surprise.

It would be six months before the clouds lifted in my head. I went to bed on Sunday night, August 17th, 2017, still as confused as I had been the morning I collapsed. I woke up on Monday the 18th, and it was like someone had washed the windscreen in my mind and I could finally see through it. The best way I can describe it is that it's like going to an ophthalmologist and needing glasses. You didn't know how bad your eyes were until you put on your new prescription lenses and everything came into view. My brain had a new prescription and I could see sharp once again. This was nearly the person I lost all those months ago on that floor in the attic and now he was back, for the most part. The contrast was incredible and I felt a little overwhelmed.

The next big step in my recovery was going to be having my heart repaired. I was assigned to a specialist surgeon in the Royal Victoria Hospital in Belfast, Colum Owens. When asked who was going to be doing the surgery, a colleague of mine at work told his brother, an NHS Cardiologist, who was doing it. His brother told him that Dr. Owens was the "rock-star" of heart surgeons in Northern Ireland, which was obviously comforting. Of course, there were possible complications, many complications, and what happened to Tim was still fresh in my mind. Roisin and I were obviously concerned and we knew that even the most routine surgery, particularly around the heart, was delicate. We put our trust in the Surgical team that they would deliver me safely out the other side. The surgery was to take place in November, nine months after the stroke. It had to be done and I knew that it would make me healthier in the long run.

FIVE YEARS RUNNING

I didn't race at all in 2017. I did, however, take part in my fifth consecutive Dublin City Marathon on October 29, 2017, as a pacer for a friend running her first marathon. My head was clear and I knew that I could manage the distance as long as I kept the pace in check. We got our long runs in and kept up our weekly mileage so the training was in place to complete the race, but it had been a year since my last one and all the gratitude and clarity of mind in the world wasn't going to help my body run a marathon. We had to go out and do it.

One of the nice things about pacing duties is that you usually run at a comfortable pace, otherwise you shouldn't be pacing for that time. Secondly, there is company the whole way around the course. What more could I ask for in my first marathon back? My watch proved that we ran a remarkably steady pace going 1:51:51 for the first half and 1:51:48 for the second half. There was only one toilet stop along the route, which turned out to be an eye-opening experience for my partner in crime, who came out of the portaloo looking as if she was witness to one of the worst atrocities known to man. I've never required the use of an on-course facility, but from the sounds of it, I don't think I ever want to be privy to such an experience. After rinsing her hands off with a bottle of water, and she stopped retching, we were back underway, maybe just a little wiser than before.

Our chip time was 3:43:22, coming out of the second wave of runners. We were both happy with that result as it was a London Marathon qualifying time for her, and I was thrilled to have just completed it. I proved to myself that I could still manage the distance and stand at the finish. I'd come a long way in eight months. This marathon brought an extremely challenging period of my life to a satisfying conclusion. There was still the not-so-small procedure coming up soon: heart surgery. Those are two words nobody wants to hear.

CHAPTER 14
THE REPAIR SHOP

ALL BABIES DEVELOP in the mother's womb with a hole in their heart, which plays an important role in their development. It allows for the mother's oxygen rich blood to pass through the baby's heart and brain. After birth, this hole, known as a Patent Foramen Ovale (PFO), will normally close over, leaving a perfectly healthy heart. Occasionally, this small hole doesn't fully close and remains in approximately 20% of healthy adults. In most cases, the hole is small enough that it causes no real issues and the adult won't ever know they have it. Among these 20% of adults, however, is a small proportion who will be left with a larger hole, called an Atrial Septal Defect which presents much more dangerous risks. This 11mm hole in my heart was exactly that, an ASD.

The operation to repair my heart was scheduled for November 16, 2017. This procedure, known as an ASD closure, wasn't quite routine surgery but it was fairly common and I was to be in the care of the best doctors. That said, in the back of my mind was what happened to Tim only two and a half years ago.

His was to have been routine heart surgery in one of the world's leading hospitals and it still went tragically wrong. Nothing in this life is guaranteed, that's for sure.

In September and October, I had meetings with the surgeon and his team. They were extremely comforting and I don't think I've ever met anyone with as much confidence in his ability as Dr. Owens. There was a specialist nurse who gave me her card and told me that if I had any questions before the surgery, I should just lift the phone and ring her. The entire team was extremely professional and, although I had concerns, I don't think anyone could have eased my mind any more than they did.

I did my best to make sure everything was in order, including making my will. Also, in the days leading up to the operation, I wrote letters to each of my kids and Roisin and left these in my desk drawer. On the off chance I didn't make it, I wanted to give them some final words and tell them how much I loved them. I texted friends and family, letting them know I loved them all. I didn't want anything left undone. I had read up on the procedure I was to have, and although the surgeon left me feeling like everything would be fine, it still wasn't without risk. He had done this many times and I was in good hands, but that didn't stop him from explaining that *death* was a possible complication

I can't count the number of times my brother Kevin was there for me when I needed him most throughout my life and once again, he was at my side on the day the surgery was to take place. He flew in from Boston the day before and accompanied Roisin and I to the hospital. Having these two people at my side made the whole thing that much easier to take on. I'm not sure I was able to express this sentiment at the time, but they knew, and if they didn't, they certainly do now.

The 16th arrived and we drove to Belfast early in the morning for my appointment. I was admitted into the Cardiac ward in the Royal Victoria Hospital and filled in most of the paperwork, changed into my hospital gown, and prepared for the operation. As I was lying up in the ward, a nurse came in to take care of a few things. She told Roisin and Kevin that it would be a while before I would be taken in, and they had plenty of time to go and grab a coffee, which they did. About 15 minutes later, the nurse announced the time had come. I was wheeled out to the hallway and parked up while they asked me to provide one last signature on one last form. This was moving along faster than any of us thought. The hospital staff were wheeling me into the operating theatre when Roisin came running to the bed, a little teary eyed. She thought she was going to miss seeing me one last time with my *holey* heart. She caught me just in time, wished me luck, and we exchanged all the lovey-dovey emotions. It may sound like I'm being casual about it now, but I was quiet and mentally preparing for this, which probably made me seem distant to Roisin. In fact, reality was just kicking in and I suppose I was a bit stoic more than anything. I had made all my preparations and anything that was going to happen was out of our hands now.

There was a team of four doctors in the room and a couple of nurses. We had some little chit-chat and the anaesthesiologist said a few things, I can't honestly recall, but it was to ease my mind a wee bit. He then asked me to count back from ten. I think I got to eight and that's the last I remember of the oper-ating room.

During my procedure, the surgeon made an incision in the

main artery in my right groin area and inserted a catheter, snaking it all the way up into the middle of my heart. Inside this tube was a collapsed disc made from nickel titanium mesh. This 15mm Oculatek disc was inserted through the hole in my heart, extracted, and it expanded. The surgeon then pulled the tube back slightly, which then extracted the second half of this disk. It expanded on the near side of the hole. The two sides of the disc were then cinched together and attached to the wall of the septum separating the two chambers. Over the course of the following weeks and months, the heart tissue grows over this metal mesh and creates a fully closed and more efficient heart.

I woke up a while later in an open ward with five other patients recovering from one procedure or another. Obviously, I was a bit dazed and confused at first, but in a short time I came around. Before long, Roisin and Kevin were able to come in and visit. I didn't see the doctor until the following morning but I got word that everything went well and they were all pleased with the outcome. Upon close inspection, I had a small incision about 1cm in length in my right groin and a massive bruise around it had already started to appear.

The evening was mostly comfortable but a little loud, due in no small part to one of my roommates snoring for Ireland. I actually recorded it on my phone because I didn't think anyone would believe me when I said the entire room was shaking. It was like an episode out of the Three Stooges. Thankfully, I spent just one night recovering in the hospital before heading back to the comfort of home. The bruise on my groin continued to expand over the next few days and turned every shade of brown and yellow. I also had a few days of fatigue, probably caused by the anaesthesia, but all seemed fine otherwise and I spent a few easy days relaxing at home with Roisin, Kevin and my kids.

CHAPTER 15
A COUPLE OF BLIPS

IN THE SECOND week of recovery, I began experiencing some unusual dizziness and light-headedness. My heart rate was staying quite low for longer periods as well, sometimes down under 30 bpm. This was obviously a concern so soon after heart surgery and as we were instructed to phone the doctor if I experienced anything unusual, we did just that. Roisin took me back to the A & E department in Enniskillen and while being interviewed by the staff upon my arrival, I nearly passed out in the office chair. My head just went swimming briefly and the nurse caught me and sat me back up. She called for help and I was soon admitted back in for a brief stay in the South West Acute Hospital.

I was hooked back up to all the monitors and put under observation. I was also given a battery of tests including an ECG. Thankfully, Dr. Monaghan was back on the case and there didn't seem to be any immediate danger. The closure device hadn't dislodged or moved, so that was the biggest fear put to bed. What I had was a sinus bradycardia, which in layman's terms is a slow heartbeat. This wasn't anything to be overly concerned about as it is normal for me, but what was an issue was something that had showed up on the ECG. It is called Mobitz Type II. This is something that Dr. Monaghan had found on my first stay in the hospital, but there were more pressing issues to deal with at that time. Mobitz Type II shows up on the ECG when the second blip doesn't fire. A heartbeat usually sounds something like da-dub, da-dub, da-dub, da-dub. Mobitz Type II sounds like da-dub, da-dub, da-dub, da, and missing that last dub. This will, at some time in the future, require the use of a pacemaker to ensure a healthy heartbeat, but in the short term, I was relieved to hear that this wasn't something I would need just yet. My body had been working with a significantly inefficient heart for so long, it was just going to need more time to adjust to having one that worked properly. I spent a total of one week in the SWAH this time around while these tests were carried out before I was discharged once again. I was back at work the following Monday.

There is only one final footnote on this for now. In June 2020, I had a similar issue with bradycardia. I spent another four-day holiday in the SWAH. This time, the world was battling COVID so my hospital stay was a completely different experience. The staff were still amazing, but there were no visitors and the personal protection equipment was more prevalent than ever. Everything was checking out similarly as the last time I had a blip. I had a low heart rate going in and it came back around after a few hours. However, on the first night there, as they were taking a blood sample, I collapsed as my heart stopped for six seconds. The next thing I remember is waking up to a team of nurses surrounding me and alarms going off like a bank heist was in progress. The cardiologists on call that night decided that

I was to get the pacemaker the next morning and they made all the arrangements for me to be transferred to Belfast. They consulted Dr. Monaghan when she came in the following morning, as she was familiar with me and my history. She decided the time still wasn't just right and the pacemaker was cancelled. I was kept in for observation for another couple of days and everything settled down once again. As far as I'm concerned, this was a relief. I know my heart has some issues, but the longer I can go without the pacemaker the better. Once it's in, it's not coming out.

I don't think my feelings about my recovery could be summed up any better than by quoting the New York Yankee legend Lou Gehrig. He was diagnosed with Amyotrophic Lateral Sclerosis (ALS), now known as Lou Gehrig's disease, on his 36th birthday. Known as the Iron Horse for his indefatigable career as one of the greatest baseball players of all time, having played in an astounding 2,130 consecutive games. Gehrig, a tremendous hitter for average and power, was rapidly losing strength and speed. In May 1939, one of the greatest players on one of the greatest teams sat himself on the bench. On his appreciation day at Yankee Stadium on the 4th of July, 1939 he delivered one of the most well known speeches when said the following words:

Fans, for the past two weeks you have been reading about the bad break I got. Yet today I consider myself the luckiest man on the face of this earth. I have been in ballparks for seventeen years and have never received anything but kindness and encouragement from you fans.

Look at these grand men. Which of you wouldn't consider it the highlight of his career just to associate with them for even one day? Sure, I'm lucky. Who wouldn't consider it an honour to have known Jacob Ruppert? Also, the builder of baseball's greatest empire, Ed Barrow? To have spent six years with that wonderful little fellow, Miller Huggins? Then to have spent the next nine years with that outstanding leader, that smart student of psychology, the best manager in baseball today, Joe McCarthy? Sure, I'm lucky.

When the New York Giants, a team you would give your right arm to beat, and vice versa, sends you a gift - that's something. When everybody down to the groundskeepers and those boys in white coats remember you with trophies - that's something. When you have a wonderful mother-in-law who takes sides with you in squabbles with her own daughter - that's something. When you have a father and a mother who work all their lives so you can have an education and build your body - it's a blessing. When you have a wife who has been a tower of strength and shown more courage than you dreamed existed - that's the finest I know.

So I close in saying that I may have had a tough break, but I have an awful lot to live for.

I could recite most of those words inserting different names where he mentions individuals and it would be just as fitting as if I said them. Gehrig sadly passed away just two years later, on June 2, 1941. The words he spoke on that day will go down in sports history as one of the most generous speeches full of appreciation and gratitude for the people in his life, his family, teammates, fans and for the sport which he loved.

Unlike Lou Gehrig, I was given a second chance in life. I have a repaired heart and one that is working near its full capacity for the first time since I was born. I won't need a pacemaker for some years to come. I survived a life-threatening event. I do honestly consider myself the luckiest man on the face of the earth. I too am appreciative and grateful for those things; the people in my life, my family, friends, club mates, and in no small way, the sport of running.

CHAPTER 16
THIS THING WORKS

I TOOK a month off running as I recovered from surgery, and the second spell in the hospital. My resting heart rate was back to a healthy rhythm in the low 40s. There were those friends and family who didn't think it was a good idea for me to be back running so soon after having a small piece of metal inserted into my heart. These well-meaning individuals knew, however, how important it was for me to be back doing what I loved doing. I received reassuring feedback from the team of doctors who still cared for me that all was well. They were confident that my heart was healing nicely and I was OK to run, and actually exert myself, when I felt I was ready.

I took my time building up to speed work and didn't run anything faster than eight-minute miles until March. Later in that month, I ran my first marathon, and despite a tough run, my confidence in my previously damaged body grew. Ironically, it was because it was such a bad run, and I survived, that I was convinced my body was healing. It was time I took the training wheels off. I had a desire to test myself once again, and see if it was possible to get back to my previous standard. I knew it would be a challenge. Anything worthwhile takes time and effort to achieve. However, I was determined to be a happy runner, whether or not I produced the results I had in the past.

IT MAY BE WESTERN, BUT IT WASN'T GREAT

All I can say about my first marathon back after my heart surgery is that it was an awful experience. In March of 2018 I was part of a group of eight who travelled to Westport, in County Mayo, the night before the Great Western Greenway Marathon. We rented an Airbnb and had an interesting pre-race evening with the owner of the property, who decided to sit up drinking wine with us until late into the evening. To clarify, he was drinking wine, not us. Our wine would wait until the following night. He was full of craic and certainly had that famous *gift of the gab* that the Irish are so well known for. He waxed lyrical on his one marathon running experience, when his brother challenged him to run Dublin one year and the two of them completed it in just over three hours. I'm not sure we were convinced of the accuracy of his story, but we enjoyed it. There were a lot of laughs that night thanks to our new friend, and it certainly made for the start of another great running adventure. To be honest, none of us really trained for this one and we were treating it more like a weekend away than a race. During the lead up to it, I had only run one 20 miler since the previous October in Dublin. That race just so happened to be my 24th marathon. I had the number 25 in my head and I liked the sound of reaching that milestone. So I decided to run this, even without any focused training. I figured I should be able to finish the distance as long as I didn't worry about the time. Over ambitious? Quite possibly, but there was only one way to find out.

This was to be a gentle run along the Greenway between Achill Island and Westport in County Mayo. This is a beautifully rugged part of Ireland. It is mostly on a path between the two locations with a few stretches on the roads. We got the bus out from Westport and they dropped us off near the start line in Achill. By this time of the morning, it was clear and sunny, which created conditions that were actually great for a long run.

I, along with two others, decided at the start that we had similar objectives so we would stick together and run an easy enough 8:30/mile pace and just get around it. Well, as the three of us did our thing, like all runners inevitably do, we just couldn't seem to manage to keep the pace at 8:30 or slower, each mile ticked over a little bit too fast. After about 18 miles or so the first of us decided to slow down a bit and asked the other two to go on, which we did. At about mile 24, the other runner and I seemed to be going OK but soon enough he told me he was going to slow down as his feet were bothering him and he told me to go on. If only a marathon was 24 miles.

Not a half mile after that I hit the wall, hard. Like someone who doesn't notice the clear glass sliding doors leading out to the patio and walks straight into it at full speed. That was me, knocked almost backwards. Mentally, I was no longer in the game. My head had given up completely. I've never experienced such a quick demise in any race before. I just stopped. Unsure why my body wasn't doing what it was supposed to do. My legs had become disconnected from the neural pathways to my brain. I tried to jog but couldn't so I walked. I tried to jog again, but couldn't and stopped again. Alone, under the shade of a tree tunnel, I returned to walking. Soon, my friend passed me. I still had a mile and a half to go. I continued to walk, shuffle, drag myself up a slight hill as though it was Everest. Then the other friend who had slowed down first caught me and her instincts kicked in. She stuck with me and talked me through that last mile and a half. If it wasn't for her, I'd probably still be out there. My splits over the last three miles looked like this:

Mile 24: 10:44

Mile 25: 13:37

Mile 26: 13:18

I eventually finished in a time of 3:55:22. I'm sure it was just that I was out of shape, as opposed to suffering the after effects of the heart surgery, but trying to convince people I was OK, well, that was another thing altogether. For about two years, my good friend Tara would scold me if she thought I was running too hard or if I looked in any way pale or struggling. I've gotten many such earfuls as Tara and I tend to enter all the same races. That has passed now, but it certainly took some convincing for her to stop worrying about my recovery.

As the rest of the group of runners enjoyed the post-race refreshments in the Westport House Visitor Centre I laid down in the back of my car, huddled up and shivering. I was freezing, nauseous, and sore in every part of my body. To make matters worse, I had to drive home, which is a two-and-a-half-hour trip. We managed to make it about 20 miles before I had to stop the car along the main road and get sick. After that, someone else took over driving duties as my current shade of blue wasn't exactly inspiring confidence that I could make it all the way back to Fermanagh.

LONDON CALLING

There are six marathon majors in the world, as of this writing anyway. Boston, New York, Chicago, London, Berlin and Tokyo. London is without a doubt the most popular among those of us in the UK and Ireland, just because of the proximity. It felt like I was the only runner who hadn't taken part in it. London has a terrific reputation as a fast, flat course with an amazing amount of support on the streets of the city. With my Dublin Marathon finish under 3:15 from October 2016, and as a man between the ages of 45-50, I earned a good-for-age place in the 2018 event. Unlike Boston, London accepted all qualifying entries, so I was guaranteed a place as long as I followed the simple instructions. I entered my qualification and settled in thinking that was me sorted. As the time rolled around and many of my friends were starting to receive their acceptance letters from London, I patiently awaited mine. Day after day rolled by and nothing came.

There was a couple of weeks during which I was having email issues and I missed two weeks' worth of messages into my main account. This coincided with the all-important notifications from the London Marathon about my acceptance. As I was unable to reply in time to pay for my entry, I missed my opportunity to do the one race I had so badly wanted to do in 2018.

RUNNING WITH CATHERINA

Perhaps the most significant run I've ever had took place in the most unlikely of places in the most unlikely event. In April 2018 I took part in a 5k in Cavan town called Run with Catherina, named for the hall-of-fame Irish runner Catherina McKiernan, who is always in attendance. I had been running quite a bit since my surgery but as yet hadn't pushed my body up to race pace in any distance, let alone a 5k where the heart rate skyrockets. I was in uncharted waters for this one. Although nervous and somewhat apprehensive about how my heart would react, I was also bubbling with excitement to be back on the start line of a 5k. This would be the first time in over a year that I was going to take the handbrake off and go for it. I had travelled down to this race with a group from the Running Club where I coached, the Rock Runners. They are a super bunch of people and love a day out racing as much as any club. To be honest, they love a night out after a race, probably a little more, but that's a whole other story.

The beauty of a 5k is that although you run *eyes-out* during it, before you know it the finish line is in front of you. The course was really good and started with a nice downhill which got my adrenaline pumping. The entire way around felt like an out of body experience, like I was floating above my physical being, watching him running for all he was worth. It felt great. I recall coming into the finish line and seeing the clock. It read 19:25 as I crossed the line and 19:23 chip time. This was actually an emotional moment for me. I found myself a little teary and absolutely delighted with that time. The first person I saw when I finished was a friend and fellow coach from Clones AC, Paul O'Neill. I just gave him a big hug. I didn't know if I'd ever run under 20 minutes again. I thought it was possible, but until I did, I was full of uncertainty. I didn't know if I'd ever be near what I used to be, and I had made peace with that competitive side of myself. I was pleased simply to be running and racing again. But this race had given me hope that now my heart was repaired, I might actually get back to my old self one day. This small 5k in the quiet county town of Cavan was a momentous evening for me and will go down as one of my most memorable races.

It was with immense appreciation that I collected a prize for second place in my age category after finishing 8th overall. It was Catherina herself who handed it out. Most of the big hitters were running in the 10k race, but it goes to show that you never know someone's story. Knowing what I had come through and the effort it took to get back to racing was something highly personal and, in the context, only I could appreciate, with the gravity it deserved. It was a momentous step forward in my healing process.

An interesting side-note on this race relative to my newly repaired heart revolves around my racing heart rate. On my last 5k I ran, only three days before I had my stroke, my heart rate hit a high of 177 bpm. On this night, with a fully functioning heart my max heart rate only topped out at 155 bpm. It is only logical that my heart is working far more efficiently than it used to, and this feels more and more like the outcome of the surgery was a success.

A TURNING POINT IN EXETER

My marathon in the west of Ireland was less than spectacular, in fact, it was a downright demoralising experience. I was sure it was because of my lack of fitness as opposed to a health issue, and my relatively fast 5k in April was a positive indication of that. If I was going to prove this theory to everyone else then I was going to have to do something different in the next marathon. I got back to the type of training I was doing before this whole ordeal, and my body didn't complain. In May 2018, I planned my redemption and set out to see if I could still run a decent marathon, or if I was destined to have already run my best races.

I travelled with Tara and a group of her running friends over to Exeter in Dorset, England to see what I could do. I promised her that I wouldn't kill myself in this race and that I would run comfortably for the 26.2 miles. It was a lovely, bright and sunny morning and we all gathered on the start line at the Exeter Rugby Club grounds. There was a relatively small field with just under 250 participants.

There seemed to be some roadworks along the route affecting the overall distance. The organisers tried to compensate by sending us left out of the grounds a few hundred metres, before turning us around at a cone and back the way we came. This turned out to be a common theme for the day. We ran out and around so many cones and turned around on ourselves so many times it was dizzying. In total the course turned around a cone on eight occasions, each one slowing the runners down and taking away momentum.

The weather remained perfect for me, sunny and warm with little wind. Exeter is a lovely city and although the course left a lot to be desired, we did get to run along the river Exe and through Riverside Valley Park, Ducke's Marsh, and Belle Isle Park. There were quite a few miles that were off the roads and within the confines of the beautiful parkland providing a peaceful, quiet running experience. The one advantage of turning back on the course so often was that we got to see the friendly faces of the runners we knew and were able to offer encouragement.

I did as I promised Tara, and never really felt too uncomfortable, with the exception of my feet. The last couple of miles they were really feeling it, especially because some of the course ran over gravel paths and uneven surfaces. The rest of me felt fine until my watch clocked 26.2 miles and there was a spectator standing on the side of a small bridge who said something along the lines of, "You're doing great, only 800 metres to go."

"Excuse me, another half mile?", I thought to myself. "I've already run the full marathon!" For some reason we were going to be a half mile long. The extra distance we ran at the start seemed a little over the top now.

Despite the extra half mile, I still managed to run a time of 3:15:53. This result strengthened my confidence considerably because I knew I ran well within my comfort zone and I was only a little over a minute behind my all-time best. Maybe the repaired heart was working a little more efficiently than it used to.

THE BIG 5-0

The 2018 Dublin Marathon happened to coincide with my 50th birthday, more or less. It took place on October 28th, just three days before my big day. I'm not sure what I was expecting, but I had a feeling something was going to go down while we were down in the city. As it turned out, this was going to be a memorable marathon for so many reasons.

Roisin and I drove down to Dublin on Saturday, the 27th. We went straight to the RDS for the expo in order to pick up our race packs. When we got what we came for, we walked around to some of the stands to browse the latest and greatest in the Irish running world. We then visited the big #MarathonMotivation board, where people write their inspirational messages, there was a message in black marker reading, "Happy 50th John

McDonnell - Surprise :-) ! Love KM + AMD". When I turned around there was Kevin and Ann Marie. OK, things were getting interesting.

For the second time in five years, three of the four of us were going to run a marathon together. Ann Marie was sitting this one out. I knew Kevin was training for one because he had asked me for a training plan. However, he told me it was somewhere in New England. I had no idea he was planning on running Dublin with me. This was to be just the start of it. Roisin then informed me that we were flying off to Milan, Italy on Monday, the day after the race for a few nights along with Kevin, Ann Marie, and our friends Eamonn and Siobhan.

Dublin was once again promising a really nice day for the marathon, but it also always seems to be cold and crisp in the morning, especially while waiting on the start line, so we all dressed rather warmly for the run. Kevin decided to wear leggings along with a long sleeve compression top. This turned out to be a bad decision in the end. I run cold, so I don't mind having an extra layer or two on me when running. Kevin on the other hand tends to sweat a lot more than me. As he is a bodybuilder, he carries around a lot more muscle mass than I do. So as the day warmed up, he was sweating more and more. Very similar to what happened five years previous in Belfast, he started to dehydrate. We tried to do what we could to keep him cool and watered and I traded my vest top with him so he could ditch the long sleeves when we passed Ann Marie.

The race plan was set to go out at a 10-minute mile and shoot for a 4:22 marathon. There were no other expectations on the day and we really wanted to stick together once again and finish arm in arm. We didn't quite manage that pace for the entire run, although we managed to run below the 10-minute mile or near enough for the first 16 miles. Then the dehydration started to kick in for Kevin once again. The pace started to slow down considerably and there was a good amount of walking in the last three miles. We all managed to make it over the finish line and Kevin still had a personal best time with a chip time of 5:11:39. Once again, we had a ton of fun and so many laughs along the way.

In addition to the three of us, and all our Enniskillen friends who ran this, I also had 14 Rock Runners ready and willing to take on the monumental task of running their first marathon. Without exception they all finished and achieved their goals. It is such a satisfying feeling for a coach to witness their athletes accomplish what they set out to do. This group, many of whom may have only been running for a year, set their mind on the target and then carried out the plan flawlessly.

Later that night, Ann Marie, Kevin, Roisin and I joined the Rock Runners for dinner and the room was aglow with pride. These people, of varied backgrounds, professions, and experience all transformed on that day into marathon runners, full of self-belief and I'm immensely proud of each of them. As I watched them struggle to walk and navigate the stairs, I recalled my first marathon, a little over five years ago. I knew the satisfaction they felt. I knew the pain they had right now would go away, but the change to their psyche was permanent. They earned their rewards, and joined the .01% of the world's population who have done what they did that day. I congratulated the group with a toast before we enjoyed the meal and shared our stories.

We called it a relatively early night before packing up with clear heads and headed for the airport and on to Milan for a few more days of holiday. Unfortunately, the garage I parked in the day before was closed on this, the bank holiday. The amount of hassle it took for me to get my car out of the garage was remarkable and expensive. Eventually, we got the car out and headed for the airport, but with all the American influence around me, Roisin noticed that I was driving on the wrong side of the road in Dublin city. OK, I had to calm down and get us to the airport in one piece.

IS 26.2 NOT ENOUGH?

I finished out 2018 quietly with only one cross-country event and no other events after Dublin. My body felt strong and I no longer worried too much about my stroke and surgery. Physically, I felt things were going in the right direction, and I was looking forward to a great year in 2019.

The Irish 50k National Championship takes place annually in Donadea Forest Park in County Kildare. This is a unique race organised by a group of unique individuals. They have some rules for this race that you just don't see every day. First of all, there is a five-hour cut-off. They threaten that anyone who finishes after the five-hour cut-off will only see their results for 24 hours on the official results page. They say this, but the online results show several finishing times over the five hour limit. The signs at the start line pull no punches either, saying, "No Earphones! Don't Be A Dickhead." There is generally a really fun atmosphere around the forest park on race day.

The course can be very nice or very tough, depending on the weather. On this day, February 9, 2019, the weather was cold, but there was no rain beneath cloudy skies. The 5k lap wasn't all that bad, or it wouldn't have been if I was only running a lap or two. After the sixth lap or so, what seemed like a nice forestry path starts to feel like a mountain pass. There is a total elevation ascent of just under 250 feet over the 5k lap and the terrain varies underfoot from good firm gravel, soft but firm dirt paths, to pure mud. Those softer, muddier bits get worse and worse as each of the runners pass over them lap after lap. The softest section occurs just after turning the final corner, heading towards the finish gantry, where the slight uphill pull is sloppy and deep with mud. The elevation gain is made up for with the downhills and for the most part the uphills aren't too steep and neither are the downs. But the more tired the legs get, both the ups and downs start to feel really hard.

I didn't have any real intention of running this too hard. I was going to see what running 31 miles would feel like. I ran a 28 miler in training, it went fine and I figured this was good enough leading up to a 50k. What I didn't work out was the fuel I would need to run the distance. As a matter of fact, I didn't take anything. I had a box of gels sitting on my desk at home, which I neglected to pack. While other runners brought gels, sports drinks and solid food which they took during the run, I just passed by the tables where these things were stored. After the sixth lap, I started to fade. My seventh lap started to show the pace climbing up over nine minutes per mile where prior to that most of them were under 8. Fortunately, one of my running mates knew before the race that this might be a problem and had offered to let me have some food out of his stash if I needed it. I did dip into that and had a granola bar after lap 9, but I'm afraid it was too late. Although I was able to pick up the pace a little in the last two miles my body was pretty beat.

With the exception of the start/finish line, there aren't any supporters on the course, except for the volunteers who marshal the route to make sure the runners stay on the right track. There isn't that emotional lift you get when spectators cheer you on when you're tired. I really could have used a little of that on this day. The best feeling was taking the last left-hand turn in the final 400 metres up the muddy track towards the finish line. I completed the race in 4:08:15, fourth in my age category. Interestingly, a fellow Enniskillen Running Club member and a very good friend of mine, Michael Walsh, won the Male 50 category race that year with a time of 3:44:37. He had a terrific run and was nearly three minutes faster than the next runner in our category.

As with all races I have ever run, whether the result is good or bad, I try to learn something from it. In this one I took away a lesson in nutrition. If I was to ever run this again, I would take on more solid food earlier and more often. A few more longer training runs were going to be necessary too. I also learned that I did actually enjoy the extra miles of an ultra, as there is something even more satisfying about pushing your body further and further, feeding off the pain. It is a true test of character and will. This was the longest run I've put myself through and I took pride in the torment my body endured. My heart was performing well, my head handled the brutal workout OK, so things were going in the right direction while running in my new 50+ category.

WHAT COULD HAVE BEEN

I was feeling hopeful about my running and could see positive improvements in my racing results. I hadn't properly raced a marathon since 2016, and it was high-time to go out and give it everything. For many marathoners, the ultimate goal is to run under three hours and I am no different. With a really good block of training and a fully functioning heart, I was sure that this was within my grasp.

I had enjoyed the trip to Exeter and I was again invited to join that group for the MBNA Chester Marathon on October 6, 2019. This was going to be my first opportunity to try to put it all together. My confidence was running high, my overall fitness was in a good place and, now that my heart was fixed, I was able to follow a strength and conditioning program. I was going to be ready for this one and I was shooting for 2:59:59.

This was a bigger group of runners and we took two vans on the ferry to Liverpool before driving the remainder of the way down to Chester the day before the race. It's a charming older city in Cheshire County, England. It's a privilege to be able to visit new places, especially under the guise of running a race. What better excuse could you have? We all stayed in the same small hotel and had an Italian restaurant booked for our evening pre-race meal. Dinner turned out to be a little later than I would normally eat the night before a race, but the pizza was tasty, and the company was fantastic.

After our meal, we made our way directly back to our rooms and a good night's sleep was all that separated us from our much-anticipated race. Tara and I met early the next morning for breakfast, where I took my porridge and coffee as normal. The hotel had a continental breakfast out which consisted of juice and stale croissants. Of course, I didn't know they were stale and for some reason I decided I would have one, against my better judgement, because it isn't something I normally eat before a long run, never mind a race.

The start and finish of this year's race had to change due to extreme rainfall in the week leading up to race day. The organisation was superb though, and you would never have known there was anything amiss. The course is undulating but fair. It winds its way in and out of Wales and the city of Chester. There are some quiet spots and some areas with loads of supporters. Overall, I would rate this as a generally positive race, but it's not the flat course some led me to believe.

The race started according to plan. In order to run sub three hours, the pace needs to be under 6:52/mile if running the line at exactly 26.2 miles. We were running loosely as a group of four, all aiming for the same sub three-hour finish. Two of the guys had already been living in that 2:50's neighbourhood, but two of us hadn't got there yet. I wasn't looking at the watch at all, but the guys would check in now and again and mention that we were on target or let us know we had another good mile. The miles ticked over nicely and we were all feeling relatively comfortable.

Then mile 16 hit me. I finally experienced every endurance runner's nightmare. I've never had to stop for a toilet break, but mile sixteen in Chester threw me a curveball. My stomach just felt horrible and I needed to find a toilet, however, I didn't want to stop. In hindsight I probably should have, but I decided I would keep going and hope the feeling passed. It never did and I finished the last 10 miles in a pretty bad way. My stomach was cramping in spasms and wave after wave struck me for the last 10 miles. Despite my struggles, my pace didn't drop off horrendously. It felt like I was running nine or ten minute miles, but in reality they were ticking over in about 7:30's with the occasional 8 in there.

I finally crossed the finish line in 3:06:07 and an eight-minute personal best. I was happy that despite my issues I still ran well, but in the back of my head I knew I could have, and should have, run under three hours. To accomplish this goal, I would need everything to come together on the day, and on this day, it didn't. Was it the pizza? Was it the stale croissant? I didn't know. Whenever an opportunity like that is missed, it is unfortunate because you never know when the next chance will come around. Little did I know how profound that statement was to be.

The good thing was that there were plenty of clean toilets at the finish area and I got to spend about 15 minutes getting to know one of them intimately. Before long, I was feeling myself again. When I got back with the group it turned out the other three guys I had run the first 16 miles with all had super races and all three finished comfortably under three hours. I was really happy for them and still proud of my shiny new PB.

My goal eluded me that time. Dublin was scheduled for three weeks later, but I ended up running almost the exact same time as Chester. As disappointing as it was to not hit the target, I was absolutely convinced it was within my reach. As a bonus, I now had another London qualifier for 2021.

CHAPTER 17
THIS NEW AGE CATEGORY SUITS ME

I WORKED my way back into racing shape and made significant improvements in my results. After everything I had been through, this was more than I ever had a right to expect. In a strange sense, any accomplishment I achieved was considered relatively remarkable given my circumstances, so external expectations or comparisons were not a concern. What a feeling of freedom. Every race was now simply a personal challenge and a joy no matter what the outcome.

After Chester, the next goal was to try to do better in the Irish National 50k Championship than I had in 2019, on my first attempt. I now knew what was ahead of me and I was better prepared this time around. I immediately fell into a nice steady rhythm with a comfortable pace. The lap splits are calculated each time we hit the finish gantry which is also where all the spectators and supporters are located. It is always a huge boost when passing this point. I learned the hard way the previous year that I needed to get my fuel into me earlier and more often. This year I packed water, gels and cereal bars. After the fifth lap

I stopped each time I passed this point and took on half a cereal bar and 250ml of water. It made a massive difference in how I felt in the latter part of the day. Lap after lap I felt strong. Each nutrition stop only lasted about 10 to 15 seconds before I was back on course.

I made my way around the last lap, and my legs were burning but I knew that each step was taking me closer to the finish line. The lap was just 3.1 miles. "Surely," my head was telling me, "You can do 3.1 miles in your sleep!" I clearly recall picking up the pace as I went. The sooner I got to the finish, the sooner I could stop and get on the sports massage table. The sooner I could get into some warm clothes. savour a hot coffee, eat a hot meal. I turned the final corner and made my way up the muddy climb towards the finish, with the supporters making their noise. I could see the clock ticking by at 3:50:10. I gave it all I had left for the last 30 or 40 metres and finished in 3:50:50. I was hoping to run under four hours, so to finish 10 minutes better than that was a brilliant result for me. As I crossed the line, Tara was waiting. She helped me over to a seat where a race marshal got me a can of Coke. I was delighted with my time and I stepped away to be on my own for a few minutes to really appreciate the circumstances. Meanwhile, Tara had taken a quick photo and sent it to Roisin to let her know I had finished and I was still in one piece.

It was a great day as far as I was concerned. My time was good enough for 21st overall and I was the first Male over 50 to finish, nearly eight minutes ahead of the next man my age. A little research on the internet will show that in 2020 I ended up having the 12th best 50k time for men in my age category in the world[1]. Now, I understand many events were cancelled in 2020 due to COVID, but first of all, I'll take it! And second of all, there were over 700 results that year for my age category, so 12th is an achievement of which I'm very proud. Also, I must take into account that the top three men in the category ran their 50k indoors, not on the muddy trails in a County Kildare forest park.

I had accomplished something I had set out to do, but I still wanted a sub three-hour marathon. My third attempt to run the Manchester Marathon was coming up in just over six weeks and I was overflowing with confidence. The timing was just right to throw a fast marathon into the mix.

CHAPTER 18
TWO YEARS TO FORGET

I HAD big plans and high hopes for 2020 after my result in the Donadea 50k. Next up was the Manchester Marathon in April and then my second major in Chicago, scheduled for October. I had signed up for Manchester in each of the previous three years and each year something got in the way of me running it. In 2017, it was the little matter of suffering a stroke. In 2018 it was the recovery from heart surgery that prevented a good training block. In 2019, I injured my hamstring running a local one-mile relay race with my family. For some reason, it was as if fate was against me. But this was going to be my year. I was running well and hitting my stride at just the right time. My winter training had gone better than expected, so I was excited to hit the streets of Manchester and crack that three-hour barrier.

I had one small thing to get out of the way, and that was a ten-day business trip to New Zealand. I could continue my training out there, so that wasn't going to be an obstacle. It would also be nearing the end of the New Zealand summer, so I thought I might get some good, warm weather training while there. As my trip was coming to an end, there was some talk of a Coronavirus coming out of China. On the day I was scheduled to fly home, New Zealand had put in some new restrictions and anyone flying into the country had to be isolated for 10 days upon arrival. This had no effect on me, but something was going on and the talk was that things might get messy.

The first COVID-19 related death in the UK occurred on March 5th. Then on March 11th, the first related death was reported in Ireland. Other countries were throwing up restrictions on movement and travel, but as of yet the UK hadn't implemented any. My flight left Auckland on Friday, March 13th and by the time I hit the tarmac in Dublin, in the early hours of March 14th, notice was sent around that the Manchester Marathon had been postponed. Unbelievably, this was the fourth year in a row I had booked Manchester, and it was the fourth year in a row I wasn't going to run it.

On March 16th, the UK government announced the nationwide 'Stay at Home' order, which meant a nationwide lockdown came into effect on March 23rd. Nobody really knew how long this was going to be in place, and it was obviously a difficult time for everyone. I didn't handle myself all that well during the timeframe of the first Coronavirus lockdown. Three months of way too much beer paired with tonnes of junk food was not a particularly healthy dietary regimen. Especially when no running was happening. In February 2020, I weighed in at 159 lbs (11st. 5lbs). By the first week of June, I was up to over 175 lbs (12st. 7lbs). That's some self-abuse in a short amount of time.

Although my physical fitness came back after the heart surgery, I hadn't managed to shake the bouts of depression. I continued to suffer despite all the positive things going on in my life. I had been appointed interim director of IT with Cooneen, which was going well enough, but I was struggling internally. I was out of love with IT in general, and finding it less interesting and harder to motivate myself to take on any new projects. The lockdown and my current pattern of self-sabotage certainly didn't help my professional life.

Even after we were able to start running again, I struggled mightily to get that weight off . I knew what I had to do, I had done it before, but this time it seemed harder. Along with a great many people, I developed an unhealthy relationship with alcohol. The problem was that I was drinking to excess at least three days a week, sometimes more. Overindulging on food and alcohol, no exercise, and a fragile mental state caused by a brain injury was a recipe for disaster.

The Manchester Marathon committee sent out an email mid-March saying that the race was rescheduled for October 11, 2020. This happened to be the exact same day as Chicago. It was hard to predict which was more likely to go ahead. That decision was made for me when in June the organisers of the Chicago Marathon notified runners that the event was cancelled. As with so many others, I had to cancel flights and the hotel but everything was straight forward enough.

Eventually, in May, we were allowed to run in small groups together. Running took such an effort, and all I could think was that it was going to feel good to be able to run an eight minute mile comfortably again. It wasn't good, but as the summer kicked in, restrictions eased and bigger groups could get out and train. That was exactly what I needed. On June 17th, I was able to get back to coaching at the Rock Runners in a limited capacity. Our prison sentence had been commuted, at least for the time being, thankfully. Pubs and restaurants were allowed to open back up on July 4th, and travel to some European destinations was being allowed once again.

Although we were out running in groups, and life was returning to some strange sort of normal, the pressures of work continued to overwhelm me. I was suffering an inner battle and experiencing anxiety on an almost nightly basis. I was getting the Monday morning blues every Friday night. This was unsustainable. I woke up one morning and it struck me that nobody was forcing me to do this. I wasn't *stuck*. I could do something else and ease this pressure. I put my notice in at Cooneen and left the job in June of 2020. This offered some relief almost immediately. I took a couple of weeks off to decide what my next steps were going to be. Soon, I made the decision to start a new company, Grogey Technologies, doing freelance software development and project management.

Despite getting out and running more often and having less pressure from work, it was still a battle to lose weight and to cut down on drinking. I had developed some terrible habits and didn't have the tools at my disposal to break them. There were still no races on and nothing to train for, which made committing to a programme difficult. Having a target in sight helps me focus, and gives that incentive to complete the harder training sessions. Even after all of the positive COVID news from the summer, numbers started to rise again, and in August and September, local restrictions were established in various cities and regions in the UK.

ANOTHER LOSS TO DEAL WITH

The year 2020 wasn't going to get any easier when my father sadly passed away after suffering a stroke on October 11th. My dad could be best described as well-meaning and entertaining. He had a real sense of obligation to family. Along with his twin brother, they were the oldest of seven siblings, one younger sister passed away as a child. It was always a tight-knit family that extended down to all his nieces and nephews, my cousins. Growing up, there wouldn't be a weekend gone by that we weren't either visiting, or being visited by, one family or another. My cousins were like part of our own household and we grew up together.

There was a sense of anticipation when the relatives got together because once the laughter got started, it could quickly turn to hysterics. It makes me smile to think back on some of those parties at our house. Between my parents and all the aunts and uncles, there was always a hilariously stinging response to any comment, sharpened by their quick wit and genuinely unique sense of humour. My father was one of the ring-leaders when it came to sarcasm.

As the years went on, it became more and more clear that whatever filter he may have had in the past, it was being worn away by age, to the point that nobody ever knew what was going to come out of my dad's mouth. Over the years we have tried to document some of the *dad-isms* and they'd make a great book on their own. He sure could make people laugh. He had some remarkably quick responses off the top of his head and here are just a few examples:

My mother is of a curious nature, and one evening at the dinner table, my father was telling us kids about how someone at work had lost his wallet. My mum, having no idea who he was talking about, poked her head in and asked, "What did he lose?" To which his immediate response was, "His helmet Hun, He lost it in combat! Couldn't find it anywhere." Needless to say, he wasn't talking about a soldier of any sort.

On another occasion when discussing someone we knew who was going through a divorce caused by money issues and a sex addiction, he quipped, "Hell, I'd give him a steamer for two bits." For those who don't know American lingo, two bits is 25 cents. Anyone who can enlighten me on exactly what a steamer is might help clarify a few things.

On one of his stays in hospital during his cancer treatment he told my brother that earlier in the day he was holding in a large amount of gas and said, "When the nurse turned me onto my left side, I let it go and she must have inhaled 10 gallons of prairie dust."

He never made his love for his own family obvious until the latter years, sometime after the first of his seven grandkids showed up. Looking back now, his way wasn't to show his love through affection. Rather, he showed it by never having a sick day from work in over 40 years. He showed it by taking me to ice-hockey at five in the morning on his occasional Saturday off. He ensured we had what we needed all the way through life and did everything he could to leave everyone better off after he passed.

As an extended family we had gone such a long time without suffering any deaths. My grandfather died in 1978, when I was almost 10 years old. It was thirty-two years later before we found ourselves grieving for another family member, when my father's youngest sister, Patricia, passed away in 2010. After that though, it seemed like it was one heartbreak after another as he lost siblings and in-laws much too fast. My aunt Ann and aunt Mary passed away in 2014, uncle Jim, my dad's twin, died in 2015, uncle

Warren in 2016, aunt Eileen passed away in 2017. The youngest in his family, my uncle Mike passed away in early 2020, leaving my father, the lone member of his family for the first time in his life.

He had lost so much. For someone so family oriented, losing all his siblings in such a short space of time, was crushing. He still had his own wife and kids and you could see his devotion to us shine through, displayed in his own unique way. Always slipping some money to any of us when we visited from Ireland, making sure to phone each of us every weekend and ending every phone call with an, "I love you."

He wasn't the healthiest of men but he was a fighter. He had faced lung cancer in early 2016, went through all the treatment and was declared cancer free by the end of that year. His breathing caused him discomfort for the remainder of his days but was stronger than any of us ever gave him credit for. My brothers' words from the day after his passing say it better than any I could write.

"If you were in a quiet place yesterday at 3:34pm, you might have heard the distant sound of people rejoicing as my father met up with his brothers, sisters and parents in heaven. He passed away peacefully and was surrounded by family. He was ready after battling through a number of health issues over the past few years. His pain and discomfort didn't keep him from doing the things he loved to do, seeing his friends and spending time with his family. One of the strongest will and determination I've ever seen. He is at peace now and finally pain-free. Though we will miss him greatly and nothing will ever really fill the void his absence creates, it was his time. It was a life well lived and he brought joy to so many. His trademark quick wit and sense of humour brought life and laughter to every family gathering, card game or conversation.

Dad, you were one of a kind and great dad. You did your best. I love you and miss you already. Rest in peace."

When he died, I was ready to throw in the towel for the entire year. I flew home on the 12th of October in the middle of the pandemic. At the time there wasn't too much hassle for an American passport holder to fly to Boston. But these were definitely strange times. In addition to the pandemic the United States was, and still is, in the middle of an ugly political shift. On my arrival, I found the social atmosphere in the U.S. uncomfortable and palpable. The U.S. was turning into what Northern Ireland was like when we first moved here. There didn't seem to be any middle ground anymore. Tribalism ruled the roost and you had to choose a side. You were either Democrat or Republican. You were either liberal or conservative. You were either good or bad, depending on your particular viewpoint. Having lived in Northern Ireland for so long I could see what was happening and it was heart-breaking.

CHAPTER 19
ROBOTS DON'T CRY

I HAD many long-term consequences from the stroke I suffered, and despite clarity returning to my brain on that August 2017 morning, not everything reset to my pre-stroke condition. I was never going to be exactly the same person I was before February 7, and the list of mental complaints, although not huge or debilitating, is not inconsequential either.

My memory has gotten worse. I used to be sharp about remembering names, dates, appointments, events and the normal things that many of us usually have no problem recalling. These things were never an issue for me before, but now this can cause problems. I've had to come up with techniques for overcoming this with the use of notes and a diary so I can work around it. This is frustrating for me, and everyone in my circle, who tend to think that I have selective hearing or simply don't listen to them.

Additionally, noisy environments will still send my head spinning. I can't handle certain situations when there is a confusion of sound. Loud, chaotic noise will start to confound my head and continue to get worse the longer I remain in these conditions. It tends to gain momentum until eventually, after fifteen minutes or thereabouts, I start to feel nauseous. This occurs in a confined, noisy environment like a restaurant, a concert, or a house party, if the room is small and there are many different conversations going on simultaneously. The feeling is like falling off a cliff, starting off slow but gaining momentum the longer one drops at a rate of $9.8m/s^2$, if my physics is correct. It means that I will avoid putting myself in a situation where this may occur but occasionally, I can find myself in such surroundings purely by accident and need to get out quickly.

There are a couple of slightly more amusing side effects that have never gone away. One of which is that I often find the wrong word for something. I will call the toaster the dishwasher or the kettle the microwave. I will usually know fairly quickly that I've used the wrong word, but sometimes finding the correct one isn't so easy, and can take time. This can be funny when I ask for someone to pass the dog bowl and I mean the butter, or if I ask if anyone has seen my mouse when I'm looking for my phone. These things happen all too often these days. One may think this is just down to age, but I'm probably just a little young for these things to occur so often, and they didn't happen before the stroke, so it is an interesting side effect.

The second amusing change that has occurred in me is that my internal voice and my external voice sometimes battle it out for supremacy. As we all do, we have that inner voice talking to us throughout the day. Well, my external voice has a tendency to answer him back. This happens quite a bit while out for a run or in the shower or driving; whenever there is time for an inner dialogue. When I realise that I just said something out loud, I may start laughing out loud, which only serves to confirm my suspected insanity to those around me.

There is one last change that has occurred to me since the stroke and that revolves around emotions. This one is harder to pinpoint exactly what has changed, but I'm a bit colder to events that take place. Not necessarily meaning that the feelings aren't there, but my lack of response to these feelings has been the change. On the outside anyway, I appear to be unaffected, almost robotic, by events that others would naturally find emotional. It may be that because I had a scare and I now understand that these things are part of life, and there is nothing we can do about them. I don't honestly know, but I don't wear my emotions on my sleeve like I did in the past. An example would be when my dad passed away, I took it all in stride. Of course, I was sad to have lost him, but I just rolled with it. I didn't really talk about it, cry about it, or even seem to mind. Obviously, I did, but I seemed to have lost the ability to express it outwardly.

The exception to my lack of emotions is depression. There were a great many days over the first few years after the stroke when I wished I hadn't survived. Things just would have been so much easier. I'd have a great day one day and wake up the next morning completely down. I had serious problems sleeping and suffered from insomnia for weeks at a time. On the nights I did sleep, I would wake up drenched in sweat (how charming, I know). The sheets would be soaked through and would need to be changed each morning. Night sweats were a very common thing.

SEARCHING FOR POSITIVITY

When I got back to Ireland after my father's funeral, I knew it was time to get things in my life sorted. I was sick and tired of feeling so down and unmotivated. I redoubled my effort to lift myself out of this awful gloom and started taking some simple steps to help me get past these episodes, or avoid them altogether. I doubt I'll ever be fully cured of the condition, but I can honestly say it's improved greatly.

One of the first things I did was to work on my sleep habits. I had been going to bed every night and staring at the ceiling while my mind raced. This is when all the demons penetrate the thought process. Worst case scenarios play out in every situation during this time, that in the light of day seem ridiculous. The worry and anxiety this creates perpetuates insomnia. When sleep would finally arrive, it would be the early hours of the morning and exhaustion remained with me for the entire day. This played out night after night, so it is no wonder this caused so many issues.

In an effort to address the effects from the lack of sleep, I thought it would be worth trying getting out of bed earlier. A lot earlier. I started getting out of bed at 5am, no matter what time I actually fell asleep. What I found was that after a few days, I was sleeping better at night. After a few weeks I would fall asleep as soon as my head hit the pillow. This also meant that I had the entire world to myself for a few hours each morning and could accomplish things during this time that would have previously been a struggle. One of these things was reading more often. I chose to read quite a few books on personal development and there were several I found that offered great advice.

None more than *The Miracle Morning* by Hal Elrod. I highly recommend this one as it was a life changer for me.

After a few months of starting my early morning routine the benefits were so crystal clear that I started looking forward to getting up early. Before long I decided there would be even more benefit to a 4am start. I do this every day now, even on the weekends. If I had to choose a single step that has been the most influential on improving the quality of my life over the years, it would be addressing my problems with sleep.

Among the additional activities recommended in Hal's book, and that the early morning start affords me, is journaling, which studies indicate is beneficial in reducing stress and anxiety. As I pore over the journal entries from when I first began, and compare them to later ones, the tone is so much more positive now. This is evidence that it has been a benefit. It certainly offers a channel for clarifying thoughts and frustrations.

In addition to writing, I also have plenty of time to read. There is so much work that has been done on positive psychology that it's a crime it isn't being taught to everyone. The books I've read have made a real impact on me, and continue to do so. Although I've always tried to read as often as possible, it wasn't until I freed up so much time in the mornings that I have been consistent with it.

Between the end of October 2020 and February 2021 the work I was putting in looking after myself was paying dividends. I found myself in a better place mentally, probably in the best shape than I had been since experiencing the stroke. This could only be a good thing for my physical condition as well, and thing to do now was to look forward.

CHAPTER 20
OUCH

2021 STARTED off on the right foot. However, as spring rolled around I experienced an injury that turned my running expectations upside down and the year was almost a complete write off. With my result in the 2019 Dublin Marathon, I earned a good-for-age entry in the 2021 London Marathon. I was also lucky enough to get an entry to the Berlin Marathon in October via the ballot. The only race I'd run in 2020 was a 5k in County Tyrone during the first week of October, where I ran 19 minutes flat. That was a good result for me, all things considered. I continued to train with the hope that the London Marathon would go ahead in April 2021. Most of the bigger races had gone virtual during the pandemic, but England had taken a more optimistic approach to opening things up, so I was hopeful I'd get a spring marathon in somewhere.

I was training hard and I had signed up for a 3-month 1,000-mile challenge from October through December 2020. I was stringing together some big weeks and these were adding up to big months. But I started getting some pains in my lower abdomen and inner thighs. Everything seemed to be OK when I wasn't running, but once I got to around four or five miles into a run, the pain in both areas would really flare up. I continued to run through it, figuring it wasn't much to worry about. I managed to complete the 1,000 miles, but not until January.

In February I ran the virtual Donadea 50k around the roads in Fermanagh. I think that was the straw that broke the camel's back. Although I finished it, things got much worse soon after that. I had no strength in my groin muscles and it was very painful to lift my leg into bed at night. It was painful to squeeze my knees together when stretching. Something was definitely wrong. I went to my physio and we worked on doing some exercises. Sometimes I'd leave and it would feel great, then on my next run I'd experience the same pains. In April I went to the GP as we thought it might be something else and he diagnosed a hernia. With the current state of the NHS, especially during the pandemic, it was going to take upwards of three years to get an appointment to see a specialist. Considering the events I had lined up, I really didn't want to wait that long, so I got a referral and went to a private clinic in Belfast. I saw the specialist there who sent me for an ultrasound to check for a hernia. I did indeed have a small hernia, but he wasn't convinced that was causing my problems.

I decided to go ahead and fix the hernia, but before doing so, I requested that he check the other side as well because I was having similar pain on the left groin as I had on the right. I had a second ultrasound which showed a very small hernia on the left side as well, but the doctor who performed the ultrasound spoke to the specialist and between them they were nearly sure that my pain was being caused by something else. I was sent down for an MRI and was soon diagnosed with significant tears to both the left and right adductor tendons. This was not good news. At least a hernia would leave me with a fairly short recovery period. Adductor tears were going to take longer. London was officially off my radar once again. As it turned out, London was postponed until October, but even if things went well, I wouldn't be able to get back to training until October at the earliest. I was allowed the opportunity to defer Berlin to 2022, but deferring London was not an option. I would have to worry about that again some other time.

I took the advice from the expert and did zero running while I let the adductors heal. This period of time was pretty difficult, as running was such a big part of my weekly routine. I logged quite a few easy walking miles during my convalescence, but I also logged a lot of beers and bottles of wine. This wasn't a healthy stretch by any means. Running is a method of escaping life's miseries and walking just didn't supply the same buzz. I did have my new morning routine well in place by this time and it made all the difference for my mental health. I can't imagine what I'd have been like without it.

The six months felt like twelve. I had a follow up MRI scheduled for October and the results showed that the right side, which was originally worse than the left, had healed up almost completely. The left side, however, still had some way to go and it required more rest. The consultant recommended that I continue the rest for two more months and start back in the new year. I was disappointed to say the least. I still had my coaching duties with my Rock Runners, but I missed the post run high I had been getting five or six times a week. I needed something to cheer me up.

CHAPTER 21
ON THE COMEBACK TRAIL

IN OCTOBER 2021, after receiving the bad news that my adductors hadn't fully healed and I would need another couple of months rest, I put my coaching hat on. One lasting lesson learned from my health setbacks is that even when I'm not running, I can always fall back on coaching to remain connected to the sport. This gave me the opportunity to deep dive into planning my comeback in 2022.

Because I couldn't defer my London place, I once again signed up for the Manchester marathon. After the disappointment of the previous four years' races and not making it to the start line, I was determined to get there in 2022. I needed this injury to heal and the window was going to be tight in order to get enough miles in. If I waited until the New Year to start back running, I would only have twelve weeks to prepare. Normally, this would be enough, however, after missing what would be nine months, I knew sixteen weeks would be an absolute minimum.

The plan I put together would start December 13th three weeks earlier than I was told I should begin running again[1]. I desired two things out of Manchester. The first and most important goal was to run pain free. The second was to run a personal best, which meant a better time than Chester 2019, which was 3:06:07 and hopefully run my first sub three-hour marathon. One of my favourite aspects of coaching runners is putting together a plan that suits the runner and gives them the best chance of hitting their goals. It was my turn. Ideally, I would finish under three hours, but if I didn't, I was giving myself a good chance of a new PB.

There is a widely held belief that everybody runs better when returning from an injury. I'm not sure if this is because the rest of the body is allowed to repair itself while the injury heals, but there does seem to be some logic in that. After nine months of resting my adductors, allowing for the quickest recovery, I had become sedentary. I had put on quite a bit of weight and I wanted to lose at least 20 pounds by improving my diet and nutrition. I would need to get back to strength training and build up my core strength, improve my balance, and do more stretching and yoga. This would require the next level of discipline and determination.

The first three weeks were to be extremely light. Week one had eleven miles in total, and weeks two and three only had fifteen each. I wouldn't hit the thirty-mile mark until week five. Even that is extremely low miles for marathon training. I included strength and conditioning work, as well as nutritional targets and bodyweight targets. I wasn't leaving anything to chance. I even booked a trip to the south of Spain for the month of February in order to get some better weather in which to train. Well, that was a good excuse anyway.

I did all of my training on my own, which isn't unusual for

me when marathon training, but for this race I was so far from where I needed to be I thought it best to focus totally on my own sessions and my own goals. I had a clear picture in my head as to what it was going to require, and sometimes when running with others you get dragged into running too fast or too slow or further than you intended.

The metrics I recorded on week one surprised me. I knew my weight was going to be high for my initial weigh in on Monday morning; that was expected. However, my daily resting heart rate averaged 60 bpm during that first week. This had climbed higher than what I'm used to and I'm sure it was due to idleness. When I'm running well, this figure should be between 41 and 45. That is a good indication of my fitness level.

To kickstart the weight loss regime, I targeted a daily intake of 1400 calories and this was in place until I got my miles up and required more fuel for the longer runs. I also wanted to take in at least three litres of water daily. During the first week of the plan, I averaged 1887 calories. A little more than I wanted but not too bad. My water intake was on target at a daily average of 3.1 litres. My eleven miles were pain free and felt hard. My loss of fitness was glaringly obvious. What used to be an easy eight-minute mile now took considerable effort, but I was ecstatic just to be out putting one foot in front of the other once again.

At the start of week two, I had dropped one and a half pounds from the previous Monday. That was a great start. There were four running sessions planned for this second week, totalling fifteen miles with the weekly long run up to six miles on Sunday. Running felt extremely hard that week as well, and I struggled to run a nine-minute mile pace. This was somewhat discouraging but at least I was able to run, and so far, no pain in the adductors. By the end of the week my heart rate had dropped to a daily average of 58 bpm. My discipline had dropped significantly though and my average daily calories rose to 2700. In order to lose weight, this would certainly need to improve.

Monday morning weigh-ins were going to be gut check time each week for the next four months. Week three proved that I had indeed consumed too many calories during the previous week. I had gained four pounds from the previous Monday and my average resting heart rate had jumped to 62 bpm. The question I needed to ask myself was, "How bad do you want it"? OK, it was only week three and so far, I was pain free. Those were two positives and I desperately needed to find the positives. Week three had three sessions totalling fifteen miles once again and the long run at eight miles. The running continued to feel hard, too hard in fact, but I completed the sessions.The first of the more challenging sessions were going to start soon.

Week four started on a positive note. I was down about a pound and a half. My resting heart rate was down significantly to 54 bpm, so there was at least some improvement in my fitness. This week included a tempo run, which involves a sustained effort, and a Parkrun, so that meant there was going to be at least some pace required. The distance of the Sunday long run was up to 12 miles and I had managed to complete every running session. After the 12 miler, however, my adductors were beginning to show signs of discomfort. Unsure if it was anything to worry about, I continued running, hoping it was just scar tissue or something else related to the inclusion of a few pacey runs. Despite my choice to go on, I was worried about this development.

Week five was the first week where I realised noticeable gains. I lost three pounds from the previous Monday and my resting heart rate was down to 51 bpm. This was also my first 30-mile week since early spring of 2021. In mid-January, I had four sessions scheduled, including a 15-mile long slow Sunday run. The adductor pain was evident, and when I returned in agony after that run 15-miler, I was convinced Manchester was out. It was as if I hadn't taken any time off and the injury was as bad as it was from the beginning.

I booked a follow up appointment with the orthopaedic specialist. We had discussed the possibility of getting a steroid injection if the adductors weren't healing and I thought this was the next logical step. There was another consideration to take into account. It was January 17th and I was flying away to Spain on the 1st of February for a month. In the meantime, although I was pretty gutted that my recovery appeared to have taken a setback, I was going to continue to train and just hope for the best.

I was able to make an appointment for the following Monday, January 24th and we were going to need another MRI to see the current status of the injury before any injection could be administered. However, the first available appointment for an MRI was in the middle of February. When I phoned around to other private facilities, there weren't any appointments available that last week of January. I was going to have to go to Spain and do what training I could. I suppose I could be in a worse place to recover even if I couldn't run.

I only missed a few training sessions over weeks six and seven. I can't be sure if the pain I was experiencing was psychological or if it was real, but I ran through it and it started to feel more like discomfort than actual pain. Maybe this wasn't as bad as I had feared. At the beginning of week eight, I was down to 169 pounds and my average resting heart rate had risen slightly.

It now sat at 52 bpm. I was heading to Spain feeling good, slightly apprehensive but also positive. This would be my last weigh-in for the next month. I would still track all of the other statistics, but I'd have to have blind faith that my weight was coming down.

I flew out to Spain on February 1st and found my way to the remote village of Isla Plana in Murcia. It is located roughly twelve miles over the mountains from Cartageña along the south coast. It is a lovely, quiet spot, particularly in February. The weather delivered on expectations with temperatures in the high teens to low twenties every day with no rain in sight. There was a good coastal walkway between Isla Plana and La Alhozia and a good road in the opposite direction to the bigger town of Mazzarón. There were plenty of steep hills to run and the scenery was simply amazing.

At the start of my second week in Spain, I had a particularly toxic day of drinking after a visit to the city of Cartageña. Although I do love the taste of beer and a good whiskey, my relationship with alcohol was unhealthy, and had been so for many years. The pandemic proved to be the tipping point where I drank way too much and way too often. It was a tough morning that following day. I was down as low as I had been in a while. This episode sealed the deal for me, and I decided enough was enough. I always say that I never regret going out for a run when I hadn't felt like going. Well, I don't recall ever *not* drinking on a night out and then waking up in the morning wishing that I *had* drank alcohol. As of the writing of this, I haven't had a drink since that day.

During the month in Isla Plana, I managed to rack up 215 miles. This was almost back to normal marathon training, and the adductors never really posed any further pain outside what was now *normal* discomfort and general soreness. When I arrived back in Ireland during week thirteen and had my first weigh-in, I was down to 161 pounds. I had eaten a very healthy Mediterranean diet during those four weeks and I was feeling more positive now then I had in almost a year. My average resting heart rate was clocking in at 45 bpm, my weekly miles were up and I was, for the most part, pain free. While I was in Spain, I had also made some other very positive changes which greatly contributed towards my adductors recovery and training towards Manchester. For one thing, I began doing a 20-minute core workout every weekday morning as soon as I got out of bed. There was also a 20-minute yoga session that I began doing three days a week in the evenings. It doesn't sound like much, but it certainly helped. I was also working hard to turn that voice we all have in our heads back into a positive motivator as opposed to the negative influence it can so easily become. With only four weeks until the big day things were shaping up.

Between Sunday March 14th and Sunday March 20th, I ran three runs of at least 20 miles, the longest being 27 miles. I like my long, solitary runs, and those runs longer than marathon distance gives me an opportunity to set the world right in my own mind. It's also a healthy method of practising positive self-talk.

It was on this run that I put my gels to the real test and I determined that the best times for me to take my gels were at miles 15, 19 and 23. I decided that three gels should get me through to the end and with two of the three containing caffeine, I'd get the additional boost of energy at miles 15 and 23. These were new gels for me and they contained 100mg of caffeine, which is more than the average gel, so it was important to test these and ensure my stomach was going to be able to handle them.

Then during week 15, there was one last 23 mile run which I found tough going and it was on this run I found the positive self-talk really paying off as I channelled some David Goggins. He has a great quote when he says, "I don't stop when I'm tired, I stop when I'm finished." I split this long run into two parts so that I could stop at my car and take a gel and some water. The first stage of the run was 15 miles, then the quick stop and continued on to the harder section of the run that consisted of eight more miles. It would have been very easy to stop and call it a day after the 15, but I talked myself into finishing what I had set out to do. This was such a good run on so many levels, but especially because of the mental toughness it helped foster.

I'd nearly completed my plan, and because of the very low mileage at the start and the backloading of so many 20 mile runs towards the last three weeks, there was only a 10-day taper. Week 16 was a very easy week with only six miles over two runs before the marathon. During the course of the sixteen weeks, I lost a total of 18 pounds and weighed 157 pounds on the Monday before the race. My average resting heart rate was down to 42 bpm. All told, there had been a massive change from the start to the finish of this plan and I was very pleased to be feeling fit, healthy and positive going into Manchester.

There were still so many questions that could only be answered on race day. I didn't race any events during this training block, so I had no clear indication of where I was when it came to race pace. My target all along was to PB and run sub three hours. One piece of advice I give to my athletes that I'm coaching is to trust your training and run a brave race. It was my turn to follow this advice. I was going to go out and try to keep the pace under 6:50/mile average. That was plan 'A', but I was putting no pressure on myself. I was just happy to be back training and racing once again.

MANCHESTER AT LAST

The Manchester Marathon is billed as the flattest marathon course in the UK. I've heard nothing but good reviews about the course and about the race in general. I eventually finished my training in one piece, and on my fifth attempt to run here, I would finally be able to take part. The only issue was that I didn't know exactly what ready meant. Physically, I was as good as I had been in a long time. I hadn't been in such good shape since February 2020, when I ran my second Donadea 50k. My mental health was also the best it had been since the stroke, so I couldn't ask for better circumstances.

I was going to the event with most of the same people who I ran Exeter in 2018 and Chester in 2019, including my good friends Tara and another Enniskillen clubmate, Damien. There were a number of runners in this group who were targeting a sub three-hour time, Tara being one. One of the other guys offered to pace Tara and I to a 2:59 time as he had run his last three marathons well under the three hours and was confident in being able to keep a good steady pace for the two of us. I happily took him up on this offer, knowing that I could evaluate my condition at mile 10 or thereabouts and adjust if necessary. So that was "plan A" and I committed to it.

There was another runner who added to my anticipation for the event. My daughter, Catraoine, had signed up and trained for her first marathon. She has been living in Manchester for the past five years as a university student, and is now a graduate working in one of the Manchester Hospitals. Catraoine is a terrific, passionate runner and grasped the challenge with both hands. I put a plan together for her with a target of a 3:30 finish time. She seemed to enjoy the step up in mileage and training days. This was going to be an exciting day for both of us.

We planned to fly out of Dublin into Manchester airport on Saturday, the day before the race. During this time, the travel world was getting busier as many of the COVID-19 restrictions were gradually being lifted, and the airports were experiencing major delays in processing passengers. Dublin and Manchester seemed to both be getting the worst of the press coverage. We made sure to get to the airport bright and early, just in case. On Saturday morning at 6:30am I met Tara for a short mile and a half *shake out* of the legs and we made our way from Enniskillen to Dublin, picking up a couple more passengers along the way.

The airport wasn't nearly as bad as predicted, and we got through security within the first half hour, with two and a half hours to spare. That suits me down to the ground. I'd much rather be sitting where I need to be than rushing to the gate at the last minute. It allowed us to grab a healthy meal and discuss our strategies for the race. There is nothing runners like more than to talk about running.

Our flight arrived on time in Manchester and from there we parted ways as I was staying with a friend of Catraoine. The rest of the group had made their own arrangements for accommodation. This worked out perfectly for me because I didn't need to rely on a restaurant to prepare my pre-race meal. In the past, I've always had pizza the night before a race. This time, I stuck with pasta and garlic bread. This was a change and one I had tested before my long runs in training. It took the risk of a greasy pizza out of the equation, something I was eager to do after the lessons from Chester. The other benefit of preparing our own food was that we could better plan the timing of our meal. I didn't want to leave my pasta dinner too late as I wanted enough time to digest and process before the race started.

Catraoine and I had our pasta dinner at her house and her friend Jason and I made our way to his flat where he had a spare bedroom for me. I had a great night's sleep and I woke up early at 5:30am. I showered and got ready for the race with my drop bag and race kit. I met Jason in his kitchen where we each made our own breakfast and enjoyed a relaxed chat over a huge mug of strong coffee.

The two of us set off for Catraoine's flat to pick her up on the way to the start line. I was in the first wave, Red A, which required me to get to the bag drop area before 8:30am, as my start time was 9:15. Catraoine's start time wasn't until 9:55 so she was very early, but I was happy that she was able to escort me to the race. It also gave her the chance to relax before her first marathon. As we made our way into the athlete's village at the Old Trafford Cricket Ground, I bumped into a few of the other runners I knew from Chester. The timing was perfect and we entered the grounds where we met Tara and Damien. After a few obligatory pre-race photos, it was over to the bag drop and then on to the start line location for a warm up. I did manage to remember to bring my gels as well as a throwaway hat and gloves. For gels, my plan was to carry two with me and take one of the SiS gels, that the race organisers had on the course, for my third.

Damien went to prepare on his own, while Tara and I arrived at the starting pen about twenty minutes before the gun. It was here that we met Keith. This gave us the opportunity to use the portaloos one last time and do some dynamic drills to get the legs warmed up. The sun actually came out just before the start which gave me the opportunity to ditch the throwaway sweat-shirt, but I was hanging onto the hat and gloves, at least for a while longer. Tara, Keith and I made our way towards the front of the wave, not exactly on the start line, but only about 20 metres from the chip mat.

When the gun went off, we slowly crawled towards the gantry and got underway, and it wasn't long before we were running at our desired pace. In the first two minutes, we got out into pockets of space and at this point Tara was behind the two of us. That was the last time I saw Tara until the finish line. The first five miles were up and down but after mile five we settled into a steady rhythm and the pace remained consistent between 6:40 and 6:55. The course had a few sections where we doubled back on ourselves and could see runners ahead and behind. I saw quite a few friends who had started in my wave, but no sign of Tara.

This was a typical race, with no chat between Keith and I. However, at mile 13 he turned to me and asked how I was feel-ing. We had passed the halfway point at 1:30:33. The question was a good one. I was feeling OK but it wasn't comfortable. I told him I was good and he mentioned that we were just over the target time so if we were going to run sub three hours, we would need to run a negative split, which is when the second half of the race is faster than the first. My confidence wasn't soaring at this point, but I was thoroughly enjoying the experi-ence. I kept my head up and just maintained the pace. At mile 14, I took my first gel. I managed to get it all into my mouth without squirting it all over my face, which is always a good sign. The rule is to take your gels before you need them because if you wait until you feel you need one, it is too late.

Miles 16 and 18 had the only real hills on the entire course and even these weren't anything like I had trained on in Spain. They felt easy enough. Keith powered up these hills and I fell behind a little, trying to maintain effort, not pace. At that point, I thought maybe this was it for me, as Keith got about 30 metres ahead, but on the downhill at mile 18, I caught back up to him and we were once again running stride for stride. I took my second gel just after passing the mile 18 sign, and once again the timing was right, and what worked for me in training was proving to work for me in the race. We continued on with a steady pace and miles 17 through 24 were all between 6:39 and 6:55.

I have always found that I lose my rhythm when I take on water or gels and it takes me some time to get back into it. As I was feeling pretty good, I didn't take anything after my second gel. This was probably my only mistake during this race as during miles 25 and 26 my pace fell off to 7:06 and 7:15 respectively. I fell behind Keith during these last two miles.. At mile 25 I was very ready to see that finish line. When I did get to the point when I could see the finish and hear the crowd, I was able to pick up the pace once again and I reached the finish line in 3:00:29. As I got over the line, I saw Keith along with Tara. She had been ahead of us the whole time! She had run her first sub three-hour marathon, which was an amazing feat of strength and determination. The three of us celebrated her success, and my massive PB, right there in the finishers funnel. There is a superb photo of the three of us having just received our medals with the biggest smiles on our faces. It was an unforgettable moment. It is perhaps the best race photograph I've ever been in, as in most of them I look like death himself.

I suppose many runners would be disappointed to finish

with a time of 3:00:29. I, on the other hand, was absolutely thrilled with this result. After the year I had in 2021 with no running from April to December, I had put together a plan that enabled me to not only come back and run a marathon in 16 weeks, but to do it with a six-minute PB. I was more than satisfied with that. My overall average pace was 6:51, which meant that if I had run the line better to reach the finish closer to 26.2 miles it would have been at least 29-seconds faster. It also meant that I know I have the elusive sub three time in me. Finally, I had run Manchester and it was a huge success personally and for many of my friends and Catraoine as well.

Having coached Catraoine with a target finish time of 3:30, she ran her first marathon in a time of 3:27:22. That was a massive result. We were both buzzing the rest of the day and for weeks to come. We had sore, tired legs to prove it too. As a coach, I took tremendous satisfaction with both our results.

For me, I had to adjust my plan and take into account the fact that I was coming back from a serious injury and I had to physically heal, strengthen my groin and legs, get back into running fitness and maintain a good positive mentality. I accomplished all of my goals and put myself on track to break three hours. My running journal makes for very interesting reading as I look through it, and I'll use it as a basis for future events.

A LONG TIME COMING

Having just missed out on my ultimate goal, I was determined to achieve 2:59:59 in my next race. Despite having run 30 marathons in the past, I was still learning, and I took a great lesson away from Manchester. In my earlier races, I consumed more gels on my way around. As time went on, and my fitness improved over the years, I started taking fewer. But I now realised that despite being on the course for a shorter amount of time, I was expending energy at a faster rate and needed to replace it. More than two gels were required, and probably more than the three I had originally planned on in Manchester.

I took four weeks rest with relatively low mileage, not following any training plan but just running how and when I felt like it. These blocks of time between training programmes are nice and relaxed, but like many people, I do like to have something to target and train for, so when I decided on my next race it was reassuring to have a weekly plan in place for what was required on each day.

Choosing my next race was a tough decision as it was the one I would target for my next sub-three attempt. The middle of June had two distinct options, the Kildare Thoroughbred Run and the Waterford Viking Marathon. Waterford is one I will need to go back to in order to exorcise the demons from 2014. I was familiar with the course and it is a decent event. Kildare, on the other hand, was less familiar. I always thought of Kildare as a flat-ish county, not known for its hills and dales. Additionally, Tara's family lives near the event and she was going to take part in the half marathon along with her brother. Her sister also offered to put me up the night before the run. Having the option of a good night's sleep and making my own breakfast was very appealing and so I chose Kildare as the next race. It was a week sooner than Waterford, so I quickly put together a 7-week training plan beginning on May 1st.

Full of confidence and feeling strong, the seven weeks flew by. I managed to race two 5ks during this time, both with similar finishing times of low 18:40's. As race day, June 19th, crept closer, the weather watch began. The forecast called for a decent day for racing and it remained fairly consistent as the week went on. The forecast was giving a high of 18 degrees and dry with the one negative being a relatively strong 16mph wind. Not the best of conditions, but I've often run in worse. Tara and I drove down on the Saturday afternoon and settled into her sister's house before meeting her mum and going out to dinner. We chose an Italian restaurant for our evening meal, where I had pasta once again.

I was hopeful this was going to be a special day and I wanted Roisin and my son Daniel, who was home on holiday from the States, to be there at the finish line. I actually talked Roisin into taking part in the 10k race which was to start well after the marathon. She had been doing a good bit of running despite her busy schedule. The two of them drove down on Sunday morning.

When the race started, I settled straight into my pace and within the first half mile, two other runners fell in beside me. After only a few seconds running side-by-side the three of us determined that we were all aiming to run similar paces and we ran together stride for stride for the next 24 miles. The course was more difficult than I had anticipated, and this was notice-able from the second mile, where it climbed for nearly the entire mile. The wind was fairly calm early in the race, but as the morning wore on, the wind picked up and by mile 19 it was blowing pretty hard, which made the last seven miles anything but a breeze.

Among the lessons learned from Manchester were two that I believe made the biggest difference. In that race I ran 26.51 miles, not close enough to the measured line to allow for even the slightest margin of deviance from the required pace. Although I ran an average of 6:51/mile, I was still 29 seconds over the three-hour mark. In Kildare I was determined to not only run at a quicker pace, but I was going to run closer to the line. My target was to run an average pace of 6:45, very similar to the two men at my side. The other lesson that I took to Kildare was to make sure I took my third and fourth gels with me; as the saying goes, I'd rather be looking *at* them, than looking *for* them. Here I took my fourth gel at mile 23. Although the last few miles were hard and my body was feeling worn out, I still had the energy to finish strong.

When racing so close to the target pace, there are always questions and sloppy maths going through my head. Miles 22 and 23 showed a 6:46/mile overall average. I could see at mile 24, that I had an overall average pace of 6:47/mile, so it was climbing. I was looking down at my watch far more often than I'm used to, and it was a little concerning that I was slowing down, even if only a little. Our group of three started to spread out at mile 24 with John Scott from Longford AC stepping out to the lead and Mark Raleigh from Le Chéile AC falling a few seconds behind. My watch had been ticking along nicely with the road signs which gave me some confidence that I was running close to the measured line, as I hoped. At mile 25, my watch beeped and looking down it read 2:49:45. I knew then that I had this. 1.2 miles to go and 10 minutes to do it. Mile 26 ticked over in 6:59 and just ahead was the finish line, less than one lap of a track. I could see Daniel at the finish line waiting for me, and as I ran over the timing mat, I saw that I had it.

I managed to take second place overall on a tough day, on a tough course. I hugged Daniel as if I had won the gold medal in the Olympics. It was just as much of an achievement for me. Having him there at the finish was the crowning moment. A little over five years previous, I was only starting my recovery from the stroke, and was yet to have my heart repaired. Here I was, I had run my first sub three-hour marathon with a 16-minute improvement on my pre-stroke marathon personal best, and at the age of 53. Those few years ago, I was still questioning my body and my mind. Those questions are now answered. The answer is, yes, I could race marathons, and not only could I get back to my previous standard, I improved on it.

I was fortunate to have the other two men run alongside me the entire way. It would have been infinitely more difficult to run that time without sharing the misery with my new comrades.

CHAPTER 22
A LIFELINE

UNTIL IT WAS ACCOMPLISHED, I hadn't realised how important to me it actually was to run under three hours. It is one of those things that a lot of runners believe is beyond them, particularly when they start out. I'd love to say that it was all me, my training and my planning. However, I'm only alive and well because of Roisin and the doctors and nurses who took care of me. A great deal of my progress is due to the talent of Professor Kelly, Dr. Monaghan, Dr. Owens, all the staff at the SWAH, and the Royal Victoria Hospital. It's down to my entire family, and all my running friends, and lifelong friends from the States too. Some of them I've discussed in the preceding chapters, and too many to mention were not, but they know who they are, and they include my *Sunday Runday* group with Brian, Damien, Malcolm, Rob and of course, Tara. My recovery has been a long road of inclines and declines. There have been difficult times and moments of pure joy. I have been so fortunate to have been healthy enough to run consistently over the years and The Thoroughbred Marathon was the cherry on top. I thank everyone from the bottom of my heart. I'm a runner and will remain a runner for as long as my legs will carry me.

More important than any race result is my love of the sport and my newfound love for life. I've never experienced such a period of contentment and I've never been so settled with my place in the world. For the first time I have a calm demeanour. I have patience. I'm able to respond to adverse conditions rather than react. I listen to others and hear what they are saying. I have a new perspective on those people who care about me and I do my best to not take them for granted. What is the benefit of snapping at a loved one, when patience and understanding is far more effective? I try to account for other perspectives. I do my best to see things from their point of view before getting angry because they did something I don't like. I'm on the road to being the *me* I've always wanted to be. I'm not perfect, but I'm a much better human than I used to be.

My kids are all healthy, fully grown and in their own professions. Owen is a successful Games Designer, Catraoine a qualified pharmacist, Aidan a United States Marine and Daniel a highly skilled joiner. Each of them makes me proud every single day. No father could ask for anything more. They have fallen into themselves and are absolutely amazing individuals. Roisin has been the strongest person I know; always there and always able to do what needs to be done. I hope like hell they will all read this and take onboard some of the lessons that I learned the hard way, to pursue their best lives. My wish is that whoever reads this book will find hope and inspiration in a hard-fought life. Much like in running, I've learned from my life experiences and have grown, adapted and emerged stronger for them. I will always strive to improve myself and those around me.

CHAPTER 23
STROKE FACTS & STATISTICS

I SUPPOSE it only makes sense to discuss what it was that I experienced in early 2017 and why it is significant. Most people know generally what a stroke is, but it is worthwhile to offer up some statistics and some explanation. A stroke is a serious brain injury that can have incredibly far-reaching effects. I experienced a cryptogenic stroke, which basically means a stroke with an unknown cause. In my case, it didn't take the experts long to come up with a pretty good hypothesis.

In 2019, according to the World Health Organisation, stroke was the second leading cause of death behind only heart disease, accounting for 11% of deaths worldwide. More local to me, according to healthdate.org, in 2019 stroke was the second leading cause of death in Ireland. In 2020, 6.8% of all deaths in Ireland were caused by stroke and it is to this day the leading cause of acquired disability. There are countless individuals worldwide who are left mentally and physically incapacitated and left with serious side effects for the rest of their lives following a stroke.

As opposed to a haemorrhagic stroke, which is brought on by the bursting of one or more blood vessels in the brain, my stroke was ischemic, which is more common, and was triggered by blood clots preventing blood and oxygen flowing to the brain. Generally speaking, the longer the brain is starved of oxygen the worse the outcome of the episode. When someone experiences a stroke, it is important for the specialists to find the cause. One of the most important reasons why, is because according to the American Heart Association, one in four stroke survivors will experience another stroke event. If the doctors can determine why it happened in the first place, they can take preventative measures to avoid future issues.

There is also something very similar to a stroke called a transient ischaemic attack (TIA), which is a mini-stroke where the blood flow to the brain is disrupted for a shorter period of time and is usually not a complete blockage. Whereas the effects of a TIA can pass within 24 hours, these are still serious and require the same investigation because the cause of a TIA can go on to trigger a more serious stroke event in the future.

There are a number of risk factors for stroke that just can't be modified by lifestyle change or medication like age, gender, race, and family history of stroke. Men generally have a higher risk of stroke at young and middle ages, but these statistics tend to even out with women in older ages. As for race, individuals of African descent have a higher risk of stroke incidents as far as frequency and severity. Lastly, as far as family history, this could be due to genetic tendencies for other risk factors like high blood pressure, the biggest risk factor, or diabetes, or possibly down to a common lifestyle.

There are also some treatable risk factors to take into account. As mentioned, high blood pressure and diabetes are risk factors but so are cigarette smoking, heart disease and defects, atherosclerosis, physical inactivity and obesity as well as having had a previous TIA or stroke episode.[1] Until it occurs, we never think it can happen to us. Anyone can have a stroke at any time. They happen to men or women, to children and adults, to athletes and non-athletes. Anyone. There is never a zero percent risk.

Identifying the symptoms of a stroke early is literally the difference between full recovery and a much worse outcome including death. The acronym FAST is what is used as a test to recognise the signs.

F - Facial weakness: Can the person smile? Has one side of the face "fallen?"

A - Arm Weakness: Can the person raise both arms over their head?

S - Speech Problems: Can the person speak without slurring their words?

T - Time to call Emergency Services if these signs are there.

In addition to these FAST signs there are other symptoms to look out for and act on.

- Sudden weakness or numbness on one side of the body
- Difficulty finding words or speaking in clear sentences
- Sudden blurred vision or loss of sight
- Sudden memory loss or confusion, dizziness or a sudden fall
- A sudden, severe headache

If any of the above signs are evident, emergency care should be sought without delay.

Additional information and resources regarding stroke and finding support following a stroke can be found at the following websites:

- Stroke.org.uk
- Ninds.nih.gov
- Croi.ie
- nichs.org.uk

APPENDIX I - MANCHESTER MARATHON PLAN

The following plan is what I followed for my return to running after missing nine months with two torn adductor tendons. The philosophy behind the mileage was to build up very slowly and delay the introduction of speed work. The idea, as with many marathon training plans, is to start by building up the base miles, then work on strength, then speed and finally speed endurance. Anyone coming back from an injury may find this helpful for their return to running.

Week 1
   Monday
   Rest
   Sports Massage

Tuesday
   Rest
   Reflexology

Wednesday
>3 miles easy

Thursday
>Rest

Friday
>Rest
>Yoga

Saturday
>3 miles easy

Sunday
>5 miles LSR

Week 2
>Monday
>Rest

Tuesday
>3 miles hilly run

Wednesday
>Rest

Thursday
>3 miles easy

Friday
>Rest

Yoga

Saturday
Parkrun easy

Sunday
6 miles LSR

Week 3
Monday
Rest

Tuesday
4 miles hilly run

Wednesday
Rest

Thursday
Rest

Friday
3 miles easy
Yoga

Saturday
Rest

Sunday
8 miles LSR

Week 4

Monday
Rest
Sports Massage

Tuesday
4 miles easy
Reflexology

Wednesday
Rest

Thursday
4 mile tempo run
1 mile easy,
2 miles @ 8 min/mile,
1 mile easy

Friday
Rest
Yoga

Saturday
Parkrun easy

Sunday
12 miles LSR

Week 5

Monday
Rest

Tuesday
   Rest

Wednesday
   5 miles easy

Thursday
   Rest

Friday
   6 miles easy
   Yoga

Saturday
   4 miles easy

Sunday
   15 miles LSR

Week 6
   Monday
   15 x 60 second hill repeats
   + 5 miles easy

Tuesday
   Rest

Wednesday
   5 miles @ 8 min/mile

Thursday

7 miles easy (morning)
+ 3 miles easy (evening)

Friday
    8 miles tempo (sub 8 min/mile)
    Yoga

Saturday
    Rest

Sunday
    14 miles LSR

Week 7
    Monday
    2 sets of 3 x 800m reps
    w/75 seconds static
    recovery with 2
    minutes between sets

Tuesday
    4 miles hilly run

Wednesday
    Rest

Thursday
    6 miles @ 8:30 min/mile

Friday
    5 miles easy (optional)

Yoga

Saturday
7 miles easy

Sunday
18 miles LSR

Week 8
Monday
8 miles easy
Sports Massage

Tuesday
Rest
Reflexology

Wednesday
Rest

Thursday
6 miles @ 8:30 min/mile

Friday
7 miles easy (optional)
Yoga

Saturday
7 miles easy

Sunday

15 miles LSR

Week 9

Monday
3 miles easy
20 minute circuit
Yoga

Tuesday
Rest
20 minute circuit

Wednesday
4 miles easy
20 minute circuit
Yoga

Thursday
10 miles hilly run
20 minute circuit

Friday
Rest
20 minute circuit
Yoga

Saturday
8 miles easy

Sunday
20 miles LSR

Week 10

    Monday

    4 x 1200m reps w/

    90 seconds static

    Recovery

    20 minute circuit

    Yoga

Tuesday

    6 miles @ 7:10 min/mile

    20 minute circuit

Wednesday

    Rest

    20 minute circuit

    Yoga

Thursday

    10 miles easy w/

    10 hard hill reps

    20 minute circuit

Friday

    Rest

    20 minute circuit

    Yoga

Saturday

    6 miles @ 7:30 min/mile

Sunday

16 miles LSR

Week 11

Monday
Rest
20 minute circuit
Yoga

Tuesday
8 miles w/5 @ 7:00 min/mile
20 minute circuit

Wednesday
10 miles easy
20 minute circuit
Yoga

Thursday
Rest
20 minute circuit

Friday
7 miles @ 7:30 min/mile
+ 4 miles easy
20 minute circuit
Yoga

Saturday
12 miles easy

Sunday

18 miles @ 7:30 min/mile

Week 12

Monday
4 x 1 mile reps @
6:10 min/mile with 2 minute
static recovery
20 minute circuit
Yoga

Tuesday
Rest
20 minute circuit

Wednesday
8 miles easy
20 minute circuit
Yoga
Sports Massage

Thursday
Rest
20 minute circuit
Reflexology

Friday
7 miles @ 7:20 min/mile
+ 5 miles easy
20 minute circuit
Yoga

Saturday
>6 miles @ 7:30 min / mile

Sunday
>16 miles LSR

Week 13
>Monday
>3 miles easy
>20 minute circuit
>Yoga

Tuesday
>4 miles @ 6:45 min / mile
>+ 2 miles easy
>20 minute circuit

Wednesday
>8 miles easy
>20 minute circuit
>Yoga

Thursday
>7 miles @ 7:00 min / mile
>20 minute circuit

Friday
>9 miles easy
>20 minute circuit
>Yoga

Saturday

Parkrun + 3 miles easy

Sunday

28 miles LSR

Week 14

Monday

2 sets of 4 x 400m reps

w/ 200m active recovery

between reps and 2 minutes

between sets

20 minute circuit

Yoga

Tuesday

Rest

20 minute circuit

Wednesday

Rest

20 minute circuit

Yoga

Thursday

Rest

20 minute circuit

Friday

4 miles @ 6:30 min/mile

+ 2 miles easy

20 minute circuit

Yoga

Saturday

10 miles @ 6:50 min/mile

+ 10 miles easy

Sunday

20 miles LSR

Week 15

Monday

Rest

20 minute circuit

Yoga

Tuesday

4 miles @ 6:45 min/mile

20 minute circuit

Wednesday

3 miles easy

20 minute circuit

Yoga

Thursday

Rest

20 minute circuit

Friday

Rest

20 minute circuit

Yoga

Saturday

Parkrun

Sunday

13 miles LSR

Week 16

Monday

Rest

20 minute circuit

Yoga

Sports Massage

Tuesday

Rest

20 minute circuit

Reflexology

Wednesday

3 miles easy

20 minute circuit

Yoga

Thursday

Rest

20 minute circuit

Friday

Rest

20 minute circuit

Yoga

Saturday

3 miles easy

Sunday

Marathon Race Day

A HUGE THANK YOU

There are so many people to thank for their support and friendship. In addition to my immediate family, I thank my Mum and Dad, my brother Kevin, sister Kathy Ann as well as their spouses, Ann Marie and Robert, my niece JoAnne and her husband Adam as well as their two children, Elsie and Spencer and my nephews Cameron and Derek and their partners Taylor and Sydney. I don't have the words to say how much I love you, but you know.

I thank all my aunts, uncles and cousins, you helped make me who I am today and will always mean the world to me.

I thank Timmy Bulger, you made life far more enjoyable, and you will live forever in our hearts.

I thank my gang of friends from Stoughton, Jim, Dan, Paul, Rob, Beetle, Gordie, Madan, Soup, and all your partners as well. You taught me the meaning of friendship and camaraderie. I love you all.

I thank Eamonn, Siobhan, Tara, Damien, Malcolm, Rob, Brian, Michael and all my running friends in Enniskillen and further afield, each and every one of you are amazing and I cherish the memories we've made.

I'd like to thank Roisin's parents, John and Monica as well as her brothers and sisters, Kevin, Mairead, Una, Aileen, Sean, Colm, and Ciara as well as their spouses and children. It's been a privilege to be part of this family.

I thank the incredible staff at the South West Acute Hospital in Enniskillen, County Fermanagh. I am able to continue my life in the way I do because of your dedication and hard work.

I thank everyone who helped me complete this project from the beta-readers, Michael and Tovar, the editor Ellyn and cover designer King_ofDesign, and to Roisin who read all nine versions of this before I had a finished book. This wouldn't have happened without each of you.

Finally, to all my readers, I thank you for taking the time to read my story. It means a great deal to me. The process of writing this book was cathartic and I hope that my experience will be useful to some readers and, if nothing else, I hope the story was an enjoyable read.

Please leave a positive review on the platform that you purchased this book. That is the most important step you can take to support me in this project of mine. It helps put this work in front of a larger audience and help spread stroke awareness.

You can review this on Book on:

GoodReads.com
Amazon
A Heart for Running.com

One other way to support me on this project of mine is to subscribe to my blog and follow along with the future of my running and coaching experiences.

Blog: https://aheartforrunning.com
Facebook: Facebook.com/aheartforrunning
Instagram: instagram.com/aheart4running
Twitter: twitter.com/aheart4running

If my story has inspired you to start running, I have some more books you may be interested in.
Running for Beginners: The Easiest Guide to Running Your First 5k in Only 6 Weeks

Step Up to 10k: Improve Your 5k Time and Train for a 10k

Please support your local Stroke and Heart charities. The work that has been done in these fields is amazing and your support is greatly appreciated by those involved.

NOTES

7. CHASING DREAMS

1. The Competitive Runner's Handbook, by Bob Glover and Shelly-lynn Florence Glover

17. THIS NEW AGE CATEGORY SUITS ME

1. World Ranking in 50k https://statistik.d-u-v.org/. Filter by 50k, M50, in the year 2020

21. ON THE COMEBACK TRAIL

1. I share my entire Manchester plan in the appendix I

23. STROKE FACTS & STATISTICS

1. This information was taken from an American website, the National Institute of Neurological Disorders and Stroke https://www.ninds.nih.gov/health-information/patient-caregiver-education/brain-basics-preventing-stroke

Printed in Great Britain
by Amazon

2da6dec7-7ecf-45fb-a898-532359605e3fR01